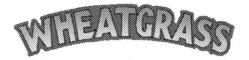

Superfood for
a New Millennium

by Li Smith

Cover artwork/design and interior illustrations by
Richard Smith

Vital Health Publishing
34 Mill Plain Road
Danbury, CT   06811
www.vitalhealthbooks.com

ISBN: 1-890612-10-3

Printed in the United States of America by United Graphics, Inc.

Reader Notice:
The information contained in this book is not intended to diagnose any
medical condition or prescribe for it. If you have a medical problem,
please consult with your primary care physician or holistic health practitioner.

For Bevil, Camilla and Susanne

Acknowledgements

I thank my husband, Richard, for his tireless work in creating the beautiful artwork in this book. Also for his support in listening to me read and re-read its passages. Thanks to Camillia for her research and encouragement and to Bevil for his enthusiasm and help on the computer. I am greatly indebted to my friend Lesley Barritt for commissioning me to write 'Wheatgrass Cures What Ails You' while she was editor of People magazine. Also for her ideas, interest and support while I was researching health clinics.

I wish to express my deep gratitude to my friend Marika Sboros, Lifestyle editor of the Star newspaper, for helping me with the Longevity and Vibrant Vegetable Juice sections and for adding her own store of knowledge. My thanks also to my friend, artist Agna Smirnoff Krige for selflessly expressing a positive view of life and sharing her ideas with me.

To John Brett Cohen, my gratitude for his early encouragement. My appreciation to Helen Stauch for her enthusiasm and professionalism in the layout of the pages. Thanks to Sandy Dutilleux for ideas on how to improve the Wheatgrass Diet regarding calcium intake. Also to Emmah Mabasa for her linguistic explanations and assistance with the identification of indigenous plants.

I would like to thank David Richard of Vital Health Publishing for patiently guiding me through the process of writing this book. Across continents and over a distance of eight and a half thousand miles, the exchange of ideas and information has made this an extraordinary experience for me.

Each and every illness reversed has been a great source of satisfaction to me, and I am deeply grateful to all those who put their faith and trust in wheatgrass and natural healing through me.

Foreword

I have been growing wheatgrass in South Africa for over 20 years, and I have been supplying it on a small scale to my immediate community.

During this time I have developed a growing technique which is simple and effective. My motivation for writing this book is to convey to the ordinary person that anyone with a window sill and a little space can benefit from this extraordinary food-source. The growing techniques and subsequent advantages explained in this book are the results of my own experiences.

I offer this information to you, my wider community, trusting in the helpful, healing properties of this humble green plant.

Contents

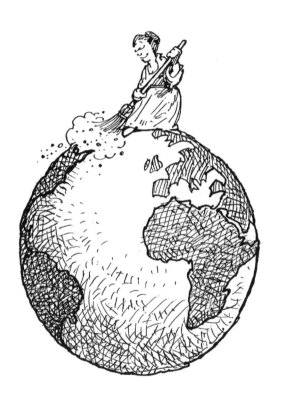

Introduction

Reality and how we perceive it always depends on what is happening in our lives at any given time. We create, we give and we receive. We make our own reality.

We plant seeds which in turn feed us (physically and metaphysically). We possess limitless intelligence.

This book is about celebrating life and health by looking a little deeper into our forests, our gardens and ourselves – a call to reclaim our psychic relationship with Mother Earth.

Plants and trees have voices too, and constantly surprise us with the incredible powers that they possess. Power to heal or alter consciousness. Power over the spirit (1).

The road to good health is the detoxification of the bloodstream with pure air, water, exercise, live food and spiritual discipline.

1

Great Health – What is it *really* all about?

A wish-list might read, "Wanted: Strong, trim, resilient body, energetically pursuing what life has to offer." A good night's rest can also never be far off anyone's list. Neither can a sense of well-being. Glowing, youthful skin, shining hair, and strong, white teeth depend largely on our sense of vibrant health, as do our feelings of security, happiness and pleasure.

It is generally believed that a balanced life-style, which includes some regular exercise and a nutritious, healthy diet; will, by and large, fight off the 'bugs', and keep us youthful even in old age.

Is the average diet sufficient to meet these demands?

Ordinary foods cannot always give us the nutrients necessary to fight disease, nor can they always repair and rebuild human parts. In order to obtain optimal amounts of vitamin E, beta-carotene and minerals, including magnesium, boron, zinc and potassium, we have to look for super foods growing in rich, nutritious soil.

What about vitamin supplements?

A team at Leicester University showed that taking 500 mg. or more of vitamin C daily increases blood levels of chemicals which signal that cell DNA is being damaged.

The team said that a fine balance normally existed between the action of oxidant free-radicals and the body's defences against them.

Popping large amounts of vitamin A may also have toxic side effects, and we know that synthetic iron can cause malabsorption and other problems. Yet in order to live healthy, happy and productive lives we need optimal quantities of quality vitamins and other micro-nutrients.

Natural nutrition with vitamins and nutrients in balanced form.

Scientists in America first started studying grasses in the 1930's in an effort to improve the nutrition of animal feed. It was found that wheatgrass provided very impressive amounts of nutrition and that animals fed on this young grass gained weight faster and were free of common health problems.

Among the pioneers who have propagated the use of wheatgrass for rebuilding nutritional health in humans was Dr. Ann Wigmore, who started the Hippocrates Health Institute in Boston, MA in 1956. She was the author of several books, including *The Wheatgrass Book*, Avery Publishing Group, Inc. 1985. Many notable doctors and research scientists have given wheatgrass the 'green light' for its ability to improve health.

Wheatgrass, which is the young grass of the wheat plant, starts its life cycle as a result of germination or the sprouting process. When a wheat kernel is left to soak for

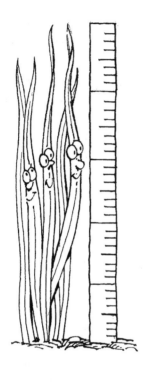

about 14 hours, drained, and then allowed to sprout for another few days, the roots become very active as they search for nutrients. When planted into covered seed trays containing optimal soil, young pale-yellow blades form at about this time and grow inches tall in a matter of days. In order for the blades to chlorophyllate, the covers are removed on the third or fourth day. By day seven (in summer), the grass is about seven or more inches tall, dark green in colour and loaded with a wide spectrum of nutrients. Wheatgrass is often harvested at this stage of its development.

Although this 7-day old grass contains many important nutrients and chlorophyll, nutrient readings are highest when the plant is about 30 days old. At this time a notch forms in the stem which signals a new level in the plant's development. Healthy 30-day old grass fares best when grown in high quality organic soil in an open sunlit field.

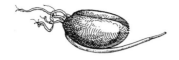

Some changes that occur in the early life of the wheat plant

"The vitamin content of the seed increases tremendously when sprouted. Depending on the seed, optimum vitamin content generally occurs from 50 to 96 hours after it begins to germinate. Sprouts are an exceptionally good source of vitamin C and B and a good source of vitamin A and E", says Viktoras Kulvinskas in *Survival into the 21st Century*, OMango D'Press, 1975.

Sprouting produces a powerhouse of mineral activity. "The grain of wheat is even more nutritious when it has been sprouted. Its calcium increases from 45 to 72 mg, its phosphorus from 423 to 1050 mg, magnesium from 133 to 343 mg. Sprouting also gives rise to the formation of vitamin C and activates certain diastases enzymes that were already present in a potential state" (1).

The sprouting process is a miracle of nature. Without it, we would have no life. Germination changes the inert seed into an active, living plant. Many of these changes create a food which is virtually pre-digested and can easily be assimilated into the body.

Anti-oxidant activity increases in wheat sprouts and young grass as well: these include traces of beta-carotene (provitamin A), vitamins C and E. Provitamin A, supplied in wheatgrass juice, is about as much as dark green varieties of lettuce (" but three times more than iceberg") (2). Dr. C. W. Baily of the University of Minnesota disclosed that vitamin C value in wheatgrass increased by 600% during the first few days of germination. Ruth Bircher, author of *Eating Your Way to Health*, Faber and Faber Limited, 1961, informs us that 70-75 mg. Vitamin C is found in 100 gm. of germinated cereal grains.

Alkaline minerals, calcium and potassium are produced during this time, which helps ensure that wheatgrass is an alkaline-forming food. The young, healthy grass also includes minerals such as zinc, boron, molydenum and magnesium, which we are told by Parris Kid, Ph.D., is very limited in even the best-structured diets.

In four days of sprouting the vitamin E content of wheat increases 300%. Some of the vitamin B-complex components increase from 20% to 600% (3).

*The formation of *amino acids, chlorophyll and enzymes* also occur during the early life of the wheat plant.

E is for Energy, E is for Enzyme

Enzymes are important biological catalysts which are fundamentally necessary for life processes. Life cannot be sustained without enzymes. According to Daniel Reid, author of *The Tao of Health, Sex and Longevity*, Simon and Schuster, 1989, "...enzymes are far more than mere catalysts in the conventional chemical sense of the word. One of America's leading authorities on enzymes, Dr. Edward Howell, supported by over 50 years of clinical experience

6

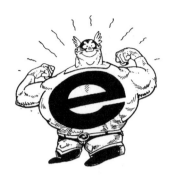

in the field, wrote in a 1979 issue of *Healthview Newsletter*,

"Catalysts are only inert substances. They possess none of the life energy we find in enzymes. For instance, enzymes give off a kind of radiation when they work. This is not true of catalysts."

Do enzymes possess creative life-energy? Reid, in the above mentioned book, notes that a Taoist physician in Taipei commented (on Dr. Howell's observation) that the radiation taking place could be detected by advanced adepts who had developed the ability to see Chi at work. This suggests that enzymes do indeed possess creative life-energy.

Chi is akin to the Indian term Prana. This *ideal* energy module or principle bursts with primal, vital energy and makes life possible. According to many Oriental philosophies, this 'dynamo' animates all life and empty spaces as well. Interstellar space is subjected to factors such as cosmic rays and interstellar winds. Our earth is constantly bombarded by these rays as well as the energy and light from the sun. This flow connects us to the 'universe at large'. The laws of nature pulsate along a cyclical rhythm, and Chi, which can be experienced as the descent of 'drops of light' into material reality, varies under certain conditions. High mountain tops, sunlit pools and early morning sunlight are but a few instances of greater amounts of Chi present in the environment. Plants are especially equipped to convert Chi or 'drops of light' into a form suitable for our assimilation. Molecules of certain pigments have the ability to absorb this energy and adapt it to the chemical needs of the plant. In *The Science of Life*, Harper and Row, Publishers, Inc., 1977, Robert Day Allen writes, "When photons of light strike the molecules of such pigments, their energy is transferred to certain electrons within the molecules. These electrons are said to be in an "excited state", and they assume a position with a higher energy content within the molecule. The movement of these electrons from one position to another represents a form of electrical energy. The chlorophyll molecule, because of its ability to transform light energy to electrical energy, is called **a biological photoelectric energy-transducing molecule.**"

We know that we can't do without enzymes. In fact, every chemical reaction taking place in the body is only made possible by enzyme action. We would not be able to think, see or dream without them. We have a limited store of enzymes (our personal store is referred to as indigenous enzymes). These are used up in processes such as cell respiration, digestion and blood cleansing. Other factors, such as illness, sweating, etc., can also lower enzyme count.

Low enzyme levels are associated with chronic disease and old age. Fortunately, exogenous enzymes found in wheatgrass juice can extend our enzyme potential! (4). Dr. Howell estimated (according to studies with rats) that diets deficient in enzymes cause a 30% reduction in life span. This could mean that an enzyme-rich diet could extend the human life span by 20% or more.

Where we get enzymes

Enzymes are heat-sensitive biochemical dynamos. They break down at temperatures in excess of approximately 106-130 degrees F, so we won't find them in cooked foods.

Avocado, banana and mango are rich natural sources. Wheatgrass has a high enzyme content which boosts the system by enriching and cleansing the blood, removing wastes, attacking viruses and enhancing digestion. 1946 Nobel Prize winner, Dr. James B. Sumner, claims that the tired run-down 'middle age' feeling is due to diminished enzymes (5). David Locke explains that enzymes are catalysts of the chemistry of life and play an important role in metabolism (6).

Amino Acids

Amino acids are molecules which are fundamentally necessary for all living organisms. More than half of the body's dry weight is made up of amino acids. Chains of amino acids attach to each other and form protein molecules. They are the building blocks vital for processes as diverse as cell regeneration and the building of organs, blood cells and muscle tissue. "Together, enzymes and amino acids are responsible for cell renewal and a huge array of diverse functions from the creation of hormones to building of muscles, blood and organs" (7). The foods we eat should supply all of the essential amino acids.

Dr. E. Pfeiffer, a biodynamic agricultural researcher, proved that on the 8th day of growth, all essential and 17 total amino acids are present in wheatgrass.

Eight essential Amino Acids:

*Lysine
*Isoleucine
*Leucine
*Tryptophane
*Phenylalanine
*Threonine
*Valine
*Methionine

Other Amino Acids in Wheatgrass:

*Glutamic acid
*Glycine
*Tyrocine
*Histidine
*Alanine
*Arginine
*Aspartic acid
*Serine
*Proline

Chlorophyll

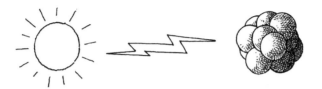

Chlorophyll constitutes 70% of the solute in wheat-grass and has been extensively tested for its extraordinary healing powers. This green 'life blood' of the plant draws its energy from the light of the sun and has the ability to infuse our bloodstream with healing and regeneration. Light particles transfer energy during the process of photo-synthesis. Sun-rays filter through the tissues of the plant and release their photons which are gradually absorbed and stored within the atoms of the plant.

Drinking freshly expressed wheatgrass juice may be our link to this primary energy source – an infusion of sun-energy may be the reason for the light "sparkling" sensation so often reported by many individuals using wheatgrass.

Benefits of Chlorophyll

The following are but a few of the benefits of this "liquid sunlight":

Stimulates tissue growth and cell regeneration. Doctors at Temple University in Philadelphia discovered that the green solution seemed to thicken and strengthen the cell

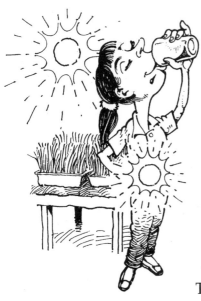

wall of animals.

Wheatgrass pulp, which is the residue-after-juicing, can be used as a topical application. Simply rub it on the body and leave it on for 20 minutes or so before a shower. As a holistic wheatgrass practitioner, I have found the pulp to be beneficial for tightening older skin and giving it a glow! Given time, it is effective in helping to remove freckles, wrinkles and other blemishes. The pulp also contains many excellent anti-radiation and anti-inflammatory properties. In my many years of experience with wheatgrass, I have witnessed the dramatic healing of many skin conditions including the soothing and healing of sunburn, radiated skin, dry skin conditions and the healing of wounds. It also aids the healing of gum problems (pyorrhoea) by stimulating and regenerating diseased tissue. It is not advisable to try this after surgery when it could stimulate the blood flow into the area.

* *Chlorophyll has proven to be therapeutically effective in a wide range of disorders.* These include: deep internal infections, such as sinusitis, osteomyelitis, pyorrhoea, peritonitis, gastric ulcers; as well as chronic diseases such as

anaemia, arteriosclerosis, and mental depression.

"In July 1940 the first comprehensive report on the therapeutic use of chlorophyll was published in the American Journal of Surgery. Under these auspices, and with testimonials by many distinguished doctors, the green pigment was described as an important and effective drug".

For mental depression, dish up sunlight. Chlorophyll is the first product of light and therefore contains more light information and energy than any other element. Wheatgrass has an uplifting effect on the mental and emotional processes and can be consumed without toxic effects.

Improves varicose veins and many skin disorders. According to the American Journal of Surgery (1940), 1200 cases, ranging from deep internal infections such as brain ulcer and peritonitis to skin disorders had been treated using chlorophyll and were 'discharged as cured'.

For more information on chlorophyll read *Survival into the 21st Century* by Viktoras Kulvinskas.

Oxytherapy and Wheatgrass

Oxytherapy is being used around the world as an alternative treatment to cure a variety of illnesses from AIDS to the common cold. It includes ozone therapy, ionization, hyperbolic oxygen, stabilized oxygen and the use of hydrogen peroxide. Treatments range from ozone steam saunas to injections of ozone gas into muscles, joints and tumors. Creams, eyedrops and eardrops are available, supplying many strengths of oxygen containing substances (8).

The success behind oxytherapy lies in the fact that most viruses cannot survive in oxygen-rich environments. However, oxytherapy has its downside; for example, hydrogen peroxide is extremly acidic and drinking it in time causes the lining of the stomach to become raw and bleed (9). In Oxytherapy, the substances to bring about this state tend to acidify the body. In wheatgrass therapy, the body tends to be restored to its natural alkaline state.

The *alkaline* minerals in wheatgrass make this a very effective organic solution. Apart from its high quality chlorophyll, wheatgrass contains beneficial enzymes, which are said to behave in a similar way to spark plugs in an automobile. They are the elusive 'stuff of life', without which plants, animals and humans would be unable to function.

"Wheatgrass juice contains oxygen. Oxygen is vital to many body processes: it stimulates digestion (the oxidation of food), clearer thinking (the brain utilizes 25 percent of bodily oxygen supply), and protective oxygenation of the blood (a defense against anaerobic bacteria). It also promotes better circulation of the blood, ultimately nourishing every cell in the body" (10).

Other Benefits of Wheatgrass

* *Deodorizes*. Wheatgrass pulp rubbed onto the skin will freshen and revitalize it. It will also remove unpleasant

odors wherever it is applied. For fresh breath, gargle with a small amount of wheatgrass juice and herbs. Cut a small handful of wheatgrass off at the root and wash. Blend and strain with any edible herbs that you may have available, such as a stalk of peppermint, a few mint leaves, a stalk of thyme or a parsley leaf. You can also brush the back of your tongue with a toothbrush soaked in the juice.

* *Wheatgrass is a great boon for vegetarians as it contains the elusive vitamin B12.* This vitamin, folic acid, iron and other nutrients contained in the young grass make wheatgrass an excellent remedy for anaemia and other blood disorders.

* *Wheatgrass contains vitamin B17 (laetrile).* This vitamin, which is also present in apricot kernels, was co-discovered by Ernst T. Krebs, Jr. and his father. Anecdotal evidence supports the view that B17 is effective in the fight against some cancers.

Super Oxide Dismutase (SOD) is abundant in Wheatgrass. SOD, with other enzymes and micro-nutrients found in wheatgrass, assists in the break-down of large toxic molecules housed in the system, metabolizing and eliminating them. They help fight free-radicals and add ammunition in the fight against the aging process. The active enzymes are bio-available in fresh wheatgrass pulp. Carotenes in the pulp also protect the skin cells from UV radiation.

* *Drink a glass of wheatgrass juice after exercising, it will help your body recover more quickly!*

* *Suppresses appetite.* A glass of wheatgrass juice gives you almost all of the 102 known elements (that is, if it is grown in optimal organic soil). It is a *complete food!*

A glass of wheatgrass juice can be used to replace a meal. It provides a quick energy boost and a sense of mental and spiritual well-being and stamina. Many people have reported feeling free from hunger for long periods of time after drinking wheatgrass. This may be due to the appetite center in the brain shutting down once the body has managed to ingest all its nutrient requirements.

Protects against pollution. Yoshihidi Hagiwara, M.D., working with Japanese scientists, found that the amino acids and enzymes in young grass plants deactivated the carcinogenic and mutagenic effects of 3,4 benzpyrene. This is a substance found in charcoal-broiled meats and smoked fish. Toxicity of diverse nitrogen compounds found in automobile exhaust fumes have also been shown to be neutralized by enzymes in grasses. "According to Tsuneo Kada, director of the Japan Research Centre of Genetics, these tests show that grasses have a wider range of metabolic activity than animals and humans, and are capable of more efficient neutralization and detoxification of certain pollutants", as cited in *The Wheatgrass Book* by Ann Wigmore.

On the subject of pollution, it is interesting to note that engineers are presently designing bio-degradable wheat fibre containers to replace plastic ones. In an article entitled "Wonderful Wheat", You Magazine (SA), 17 June 1999, the author notes "It's also an extremely environmentally friendly product, which explains why it's increasingly being used in products other than foods." According to the same article, French scientists have developed a wheat-based abrasive for rust removal on airplanes. It is said to be non-damaging to the brittle surface. Wheat is currently manufactured in the cosmetic industry as nourishing and exfoliation creams. Wheat-based hair products spruce up damaged hair. See chapter 7 on how to make your own Wheatgrass Hair Mousse.

* *A regular supply of fresh wheatgrass will help to purify our water supplies.* A Weigh-Less Water Update in the June 1999 issue of Health Talk informs us that "The American Academy of Microbiology has stated in a report that access to clean, safe water can no longer be taken for granted. Water quality it says, is threatened throughout the world, including the United States.

.... Burgeoning populations, aging sewer systems, environmental pollution, and growing resistance of micro-organisms to water treatment chemicals are among problems cited by the academy in its report."

Problems facing our water supplies are chemicals, metals and infectious diseases. In 'The Wheatgrass Book', Ann Wigmore explains an experiment done for her by Dr. G.H. Earp Thomas of the Bloomfield Laboratories in High Bridge, NJ whereby he placed a small amount of wheat-grass juice in a jar of regular tap water and then tested for fluoride and other chemicals present in the water. His conclusion to the experiment was that "Fluorine rapidly combines with calcium phosphate and other kinetic elements to lose its toxic properties, and harden teeth and bones. That is why fresh grass would act as a catalyst to speedily change the acid fluorine into a beneficial component with a positive reaction. By using wheatgrass, which is comparatively rich in calcium phosphate, it would remove any free fluoric acid and change its negative charge to an alkaline calcium phosphate fluoride combination with a positive reaction" (11). Ann Wigmore's reaction to this experiment was, "I was amazed. Not only did wheatgrass neutralize the toxic effect of fluorine, but it converted it into an ally in maintaining healthy bones and teeth!" Her advice is to drink pure spring water or filtered water. If these are unobtainable, then pour a little wheatgrass juice into regular tap water to make it more healthful.

You can also add a small bunch of wheatgrass to your water filter. Replace it every day as the grass loses its enzymes and other properties after a period of time. A few stalks of wheatgrass added to your fridge water will improve its quality. Wash any store-bought vegetables and fruit in water containing a little wheatgrass pulp or a few wheatgrass blades.

* *Waste-elimination.* Wheatgrass effectively assists in the process of waste elimination, replenishing micro-nutrients which play a role in the neutralizing of the released poison. Pollution and certain foods create antigens which may destroy many of our digestive enzymes. Wheatgrass

can rebuild these by correcting the acid-alkaline balance of the body, enhancing digestion and elimination.

* *Wheatgrass assists in balancing the body.* The young wheat plant, when grown in optimal, organic soil, supplies the body with a super formula, harmoniously mixed in a balanced way. Studies have shown that the element boron is an essential factor in calcium's absorption into the body. Calcium helps the system with a number of important functions: fighting off disease, maintaining proper cell activities, and the maintenance of strong teeth and bones, says Dr. H.C. Vogel in *The Nature Doctor*. Fortunately valuable minerals, including calcium, boron and magnesium, are well-supplied in healthy wheatgrass and easily assimilated into the body.

Magnesium, which is the central atom of the chlorophyll molecule, aids calcium and other elements to be absorbed by the bones [12]. Soil should be tested when food is grown on a large scale, as magnesium levels do not remain constant. As a result, many store-bought greens fail to reflect adequate magnesium content.

Depleted magnesium reserves in the body can lead to a variety of illnesses, including cramps, heart problems and an overtaxed nervous system. "Latest research shows that we should strive for a one to one ratio between calcium and magnesium for the maintenance of a strong and healthy skeletal frame" and "Based on the latest studies we know that the role of magnesium in bone health probably outweighs that of calcium" [13].

Wheatgrass, when grown in nutrient rich soil, is a great aid in providing calcium and magnesium (and other minerals and trace elements) in a form which is easily absorbed by the body. This 'green milk' is wonderful for the maintenance of sturdy bone health and a strong nervous system.

*Many illnesses are the result of *imbalances of the body*, manifesting in a variety of ailments including Alzheimer's, arthritis, chronic fatigue syndrome, cancer, depression, infection and skin ailments.

You do not have to embark on a stringent dietary regime to benefit from wheatgrass. Just one glass of wheatgrass juice a day works wonders!

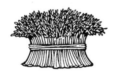

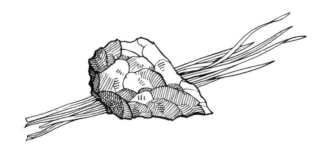

2

Grass Roots – Wheat History

Grasses were the primary source of food of the ancients. The Southern end of Africa is where many scientists believe that our 'Eve' evolved, probably in the caves overlooking the savannahs of the Kromdraai valley. It is here that the oldest hearth fire was discovered, thought to have been kindled approximately 1.4 million years ago.

The fledgling new race found the perfect mother in Africa, with her vast skies brimming with stars, and a moon so bright and magnetic as to rouse the slumbering spirits destined for creative intelligence. Inviting nutritious grasses, herbs, flowers and trees swayed before these hardy, adaptive bipeds. At this stage in their development, our ancestors led a nomadic way of life determined by food availability and resources. Guided by inspiration (and necessity), artistic expression was born with the creation of tools. The beauty of many of these early implements is staggering. Tools 2.5 million years old were found at Hadar, Ethiopia (1).

Science has made it possible for us to get a better understanding of our ancient ancestors. It is also now possible to describe the last meal of a human being who lived perhaps thousands of years ago, and is now preserved as a mummy. In all probability, this meal was made up of edible grass seeds or kernels such as emmer or barley, which, before cultivation, grew wild in many parts of the world.

Women and children gatherers learned where to find the choicest flowers and sprouting grasses. Special sticks were used to dig into the soil in search of nutritious roots to eat. Plant food was ground on stone grinding tables with pounding sticks and stone implements. These grasses also attracted another primary food source, namely herds of wild deer and cattle. These animals converted massive quantities of green cereal grasses into edible, nitrogen-rich protein. Historically, these women and children became our first cultivators. This was the start of the agrarian revolution, according to Pia Laviosa-Zambotti in *Larousse's Encyclopedia of Prehistoric and Ancient Art*. "At the end of the Palaeolithic, it is probable that a 'feminine world', a sketch of the matriarchal agrarian society, was in the slow process of formation. Women were essentially the fecund procreator. Her mysterious prerogatives favoured her endowment with the magical powers which presided over the fertility of the earth."

The mystery of farming involves a seemingly inert seed taking on a life of its own. Vigorous roots shoot downward from its kernel followed by an ascending stalk which rapidly changes in colour from bright yellow to bright vibrant green in a matter of hours. This process of photosynthesis chlorophyllates the young emerging grass. In agrarian cultures, the humble seeds, which grew so well when tended, also attracted birds. These flocks learned to enjoy the bounty of the earth people and helped propagate new species of plants and trees.

The cultivation of grasses was to place us collectively in firm control of our destiny and eliminate some of the terrors associated with the unpredictable world of a migrating food supply. Agriculture was also to occupy the attention of males in the tribe who were by tradition the hunters and flock keepers. The cultivation of cereals was the driving force which forged our early great civilizations.

"The continuing hybridization of early grasses of the *Triticum and Aegilops* genera in an area that stretched from Syria to Kashmir and southward to Ethiopia was responsible for the developement of our bread, macaroni and other wheats"[2]. The term hybrid implies a mixed ancestory or crossbreed.

During the Epipaleolithic, (20000-10000 BP) small bands of hunter-gatherers roamed and settled in fertile areas. Trade became a valuable exchange facilitated by the cross-settlement traffic that was taking place at this time. Grasses, easy to grow and store, had great potential for barter. As commerce grew, so did the hybridization of grasses. Cultivated cereals combined with wild strains and over time developed into the wide variety of cereals that we have today.

It is widely believed that a sophisticated culture developed in the Sahara before it started drying up about 6,000 years ago. Tissili n' Ajjer (Algeria) was once a fertile land with beautiful forests and lakes. Rock paintings there and in the Tibesti mountains depict Auroch, the now extinct wild ox, elephant, giraffe, gazelle, crocodile and fish. Wetter climates in lower areas brought new strains of grasses which enticed wild cattle followed by the hunter-gatherer-herder. Birds brought nut-bearing trees and the scene was set for the long-mobile groups to settle down at last. A renaissance following the restrictions of the Ice Age and floods brought great migrations of different people. Cereal grasses beckoned with the potential to be harvested.

Tssili n' Ajjer was situated in the center of the ancient caravan routes and elephant highways. These routes, trails and watercourses linked the civilizations of the Assyro-Babylonians and the Sumerians of Mesopotamia via Egypt and the Nile south-east into the highlands of Ethiopia. Tunisia, in north Africa, was the gateway to Europe, being located directly across the Mediterranean from Spain and Italy. Some 2,000 years ago, Tunis produced most of the grain for Classical Europe.

Cereals and Civilizations

Egypt, with its roots in primal Africa, was to become an agrarian-based superpower. Archaeologists working near Aswan found grains of cultivated barley that have been firmly dated as having grown from between 17,000-18,000 years ago (3). Aswan was Egypt's southern frontier and its gateway to the south.

The Nile's annual flood brought rich nutrients and encouraged farming, which in turn brought a new identity: a human type who worked closely with other members of the community in communal activities involving the sprouting, growing and harvesting of grain. Leavening, which involved the introduction of fungus to grain, was discovered by the Egyptians. They were also famed for the fine beer which they brewed. Harvesting and grinding instruments were developed. Farming also set the scene for a people who were able to produce grain reserves and devote their time to the arts and sciences as well as to metaphysical speculations. Egyptian pharaohs lived by high moral codes and were responsible for ensuring the well-being of their people. Visual symbols communicated by the ancient Egyptians give us an idea of their daily lives and spiritual aspirations.

Spiritual Regeneration and the Harvest

Religious thought is evident in rock paintings executed by pre-historic African artists. They recorded, among other things, shamans voyaging into the heavens where vortexes of energy (depicted as spirals, circles and other patterns in dot form) linked the voyager to suns, stars and mythological beings. Caves and rock shelters made impressive art galleries (for the initiated) and theatres.

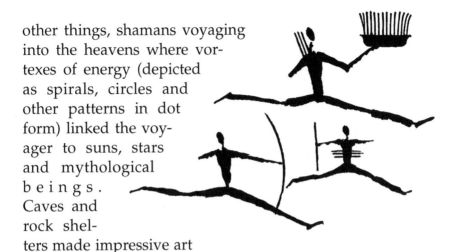

Shamans, with their knowledge of medicinal plants and grasses, were able to merge consciousness with the animal and plant kingdoms.

In the Egyptian language, Mut means mother. It is also a Zulu word for a plant concoction seen to have inspirational and magical healing powers. With the aid of these strong drinks, shamans were believed to be able to communicate with the ancestors and travel, 'in spirit form', to different nether regions.

Theatrical displays, often played out in secret rituals, were an important part of the life of these groups and a rich tradition of story-telling developed. A superb mimic, the ancient hunter did what came naturally – he 'aped' his prey. Empathy with the animal that he hunted gave the hunter a feeling of control over his environment, affording him protection and luck in the hunt. In many African cultures birds are seen to have magical powers (flight symbolizing separation from matter). Isis, mentioned in Dynasty IV in Egypt, is introduced as the power behind the throne and the mistress of magic; she finds out the secret name of Ra, the sun god. In the ancient texts she sometimes changes herself into a bird.

Isis and her husband Osiris, gentle rulers in early Egyptian history, probably descended from an ancient line of shamans. In order to survive as hunter-gatherers, humans established skills which were wholly dependant on their environment. The refinement of grasses involved reflection and had a civilizing and enlightening effect on early communities.

The wheat harvest was accompanied by festivities in ancient Egypt – a time of great spiritual regeneration. Osiris was the agricultural diety, and he is credited for teaching the art of agriculture. According to tradition, he inherited his throne from the earth god 'Geb', and 'Nut' the sky goddess.

"The prosperity of Egypt during his reign is conjured up in eloquent phraseology on the stela of Amenmose (c. 1400 BC during Dynasty XV111) in the Louvre Museum. There, Osiris is described as commanding all resources and elements in a way that brings good fortune and abundance to the land. Through his power the waters of Nu are kept under control, favourable breezes blow from the north, plants flourish and all animal life follows a perfect pattern of procreation. Also Osiris receives immense respect from other gods and governs the system of stars in the sky. So like many stories throughout history we begin with a benevolent and successful king and queen, Osiris and Isis, ruling in a golden age" (4).

Encoded in the beliefs of the early Egyptians was the idea of divine harmony or 'Maat'. R.A. Schwaller de Lubicz, *Le Roi de la theocratie pharaonique* wrote, "The principle of Harmony is a cosmic law, the Voice of God. Whatever be the disorder that man or fortuitous natural accident may provoke, Nature, left to herself, will put everything in order again through affinities (the Consciousness in all things). Harmony is the *a priori* law written in all of Nature; it imposes itself on our intelligence, yet it is in itself incomprehensible."

It is possible that Osiris and his wife Isis originally came to Egypt from Tssili n' Ajjer because he was called "the first of the Westerners" (5). Isis, according to the Pyramid Texts, was also said to come from the west (6). Tssili n' Ajjer in Algeria lies to the west of Egypt. It was also home to cattle with lyre-shaped horns. These same cattle may be seen in ancient Egyptian sculptures and hieroglyphs.

Oudja Eye

"The hekat, the unit of volume used in the measurement of grain is represented graphically by the Oudja Eye, and its fractions by the individual strokes of the glyph" (7).

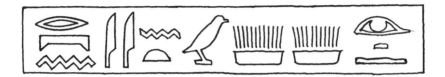

The 'Eye' lies at the very heart of Egyptian prehistoric religion and was used as the insignia of the followers of Horus who were the probable architects of the pre-dynastic Egyptians. Graham Hancock, author of *Heaven's Mirror* says "The 'Followers of Horus' were said to have carried with them a 'knowledge' of the 'divine origins' of Egypt and the divine purpose of this land, "which was once holy and wherein alone, in reward for her devotion, the gods deigned to sojourn upon the earth".

There is an old tradition associating the wheat plant and divinity. The Copts, who were the inheritors of the ancient Egyptian language and many of their belief systems, reckoned that "the wheat plant and the Throne of the Father stand in one category, and they are equal to the 'Son of God' " (8).

Religious Beliefs

The ancient Egyptians (according to religious texts) believed in One God. He was 'self-existent' (9) and "the maker of heaven, earth and underworld; the creator of the sky and the sea, men and women, animals and birds, fish and creeping things, trees and plants, and the incorporeal beings who were the messengers that fulfilled his wish and word".

Ancient Egypt was a land of vast vistas and harsh desert conditions. The 'inundations' were the waters from the Nile that were fed from the highlands of Ethiopia and that made the lowlands fertile. It was believed that the land would prosper and show healthy grain reserves when the forces of nature were in proper balance.

The reigning Pharaoh or Queen was responsible for the harmonious running of the country. The building of temples, learning institutions and granaries and keeping the calendars were some of the duties of the monarch. The Egyptians believed that if the Pharaoh or Queen lived an exemplary life they would join the company of Osiris in the 'Duat'. The Duat was a place where the spirit passed on with the help of prescribed funeral rites which included a 'judgement'. Within the Duat was a place known as the 'Eulyssian fields'. Here the deceased would sometimes meet parents, give offerings and be introduced to the 'resurrected' Osiris. Often depicted in these ideal scenes are fields of wheat. Wheat was crucial in the beliefs surrounding resurrection and immortality.

The 'Mysteries'

The Mysteries, as told in ancient writings, involved the 'resurrection' of Osiris. During the course of his reign in Egypt, Osiris travelled to the lands south of Egypt to teach the art of agriculture to the people living there. On his return to Egypt, he was beset by his brother Seth and murdered. His relics were deposited at some fourteen cult centres or temples.

Each year during the 'Month of Khoiak' at the various cult centres, great celebrations took place to celebrate the rising up or 'awakening' of Osiris.

The 'Mysteries' began with the preparation of a new 'seed-bed'. Soil was prepared and spelt, an ancient form of wheat, was planted and watered. On the tenth day of the month of Khoiak when the grass was approximately seven or more inches high and at its most dynamic, a great festival took place. At some centres 365 lamps were lit and small papyrus boats bobbed on sacred lakes.

On the thirtieth day and the last day of celebrations the seedbed was interned in a *mound* under persea trees. Another ritual on this last day was the raising up of the Djed pillar by the Pharaoh. The 30th of Khoiak coincides with the 25th December in the Alexandrian calender (10).

There is no doubt that the traditional Egyptians enacted these pageants from the earliest times (possibly even pre-Dynastic). Osiris was the first human whom they believed acquired immortality.

The ascension to the throne of Egypt, after the murder of Osiris, involved tribunals and disputes. The contenders for kingship were Seth and Horus. Horus was the son of Osiris and Isis. It was as a result of Isis's guile and 'magical' powers that Horus managed to ascend to the throne of Egypt. At one stage of the proceedings, Osiris, in the underworld, is asked to judge who should rule. According to George Hart, *Egyptian Myths*, The Trustees of the British Museum, (1990), "Osiris' response to the question of the decision between Horus and Seth is to accentuate his (Horus') role in making the gods strong with emmer-wheat and barley and thereby not to defraud his son Horus.

....In addition the stars in the sky, the gods and mankind all descend into the Western Horizon and so into the realm of Osiris. On sober reflection of these facts the tribunal of gods are now unanimous in vindicating Horus and establishing him upon the throne of his father."

Each new Pharaoh or Queen hoped to eventually join Osiris in the Duat' where wheat grew abundantly and life was ordered and happy.

The Mound Mystery

Ancient religious texts refer to the 'sacred mounds' as the first manifestations of creation. The internment of the wheatplant after thirty days, when the plant was at its nutritional peak, could possibly mean that the ancients were re-cycling their wheatgrass and understood the value of high quality soil.

Wheat was also cultivated in the fertile Tigris-Euphrates Valley, probably some 9,000 years ago. It grew like a weed among the barley. In Assyro-Babylonian mythology, Nisaba was the grain goddess who brought with her the understanding and manipulation of numbers. This prehistoric time was characterized by implements made of stone and flint, fine representations of animals, and the first woven cloths. The manufacture of ceramics and basketware were indispensible to the endeavors of the early farmer. Marking clay tablets for trade and other purposes was in time to lead to the developement of writing, which is when recorded history began.

Uruk, which became a thriving agricultural city, started out as a hilltop shrine to the goddess Ishtar. Moon worship prevailed in these early matriarchal times as it had for thousands of years. Wheat was to become a formidable resource. Fertility of the soil initially encouraged fruitful harvests, but the advent of large-scale farming was to eventually lead to the separation of a long-sustained relationship with the bountiful Earth Mother. Food resources were hoarded for the benefit of a select few, mainly the priests and priestesses. The widespread over-production of wheat and other grains, resulted in improper agricultural care and was instrumental in denuding large tracts of land. Wars were fought and overpopulation may have been a destabilizing factor. Ancient Sumerian myths relate how Absu, who was one of the oldest gods, wanted to kill noisy over populous people.

Apart from its commercial value, wheatgrass and barley were valued for their medicinal and purification purposes. Indigenous medicinal herbs also contributed to our survival as a species. They played important roles in the flowering of our civilization. The hanging gardens of Babylon, one of the seven wonders of the ancient world, were cultivated with myrrh, mustard, coriander and liquorice along with apple trees and roses.

According to C. B. Siren, *cbsiren@hopper.unh.edu*, 1999, the *grain-harvest* goddess Nisaba performed purification ceremonies on Ninurta after he had slain Anzu. An ancient Sumerian myth, it is the story of the wind/storm god, Ellil, who appointed Anzu guardian to his bath chamber. Anzu had his eye on a weapon belonging to Ellil – 'the tablet of destinies'. One day, while Ellil was bathing, Anzu stole the tablet and used its powers for his selfish ends. Ninurta, chamberlain of another war god and responsible for some small-scale irrigation, was instructed to kill Anzu for the theft.

After slaying Anzu, Ninurta visits Nisaba and she performs a purification ceremony on him. Because her special domain is grain, it is very probable that she concocted a grain ferment made from barley or wheat for him to drink followed by a wheatgrass or barley grass blend. He dined on fennel, liquorice, garlic, cucumber, marrows and mustards which were the food-medicines of the day. His bath was no doubt perfumed with cedarwood – its warm balsamic properties ease negative emotions such as anxiety. Cedarwood has many exceptional qualities: it helps respiratory and urinary infections and warms or repairs feelings of psychological isolation. These tall, majestic trees grew abundantly in mountainous areas in ancient Mesapotamia, and Nisaba may well have had a temple in one of the famed perfumed forests. Her mission complete, Nisaba is given new titles and shrines; Duku – 'holy mound' among others.

Note: Cedarwood oil should not be used by pregnant women as it may contain abortive properties. It also contains thuyon, which in high doses, can harm the nervous system.

We find references to the healing properties of grass in the Bible. The Book of Daniel must surely be one of the most inspiring stories in the Old Testament.

King Nebuchadnezzar attacked Jerusalem sometime around 600 BC. and brought back with him to Babylon, Daniel and several other exiles. Daniel and three other young men from the tribe of Judah were chosen to serve in the royal court. From the start Daniel held onto his belief in his God, and his faith and obedience (to his laws) were to eventually convince Nebuchadnezzar of the power of the God of Daniel and his people. This account is told by King Nebuchadnezzar "of the wonders and miracles which the Supreme God has shown me" (10), which involved a 'frightening dream' whereby a great tree grew 'bigger and bigger until it reached the sky' and was cut down on the orders of an angel. The stump surrounded by a band of iron and bronze was left in the ground. The angel proclaimed that dew should fall on the man and that he would live with the animals and plants, and for seven years would not have a human mind, but one like an animal.

Daniel, who believed that his God could reveal mysteries, interpreted this dream to mean that the tree represented the king who would be cut down and driven away to live with wild animals. He would eat grass like an ox for seven years and sleep out in the open. After the seven year period, he would proclaim the Supreme God who controlled all kingdoms. Thereafter his own kingdom would be restored to him. Daniel's advice to the king was to stop sinning, do the right thing and show mercy to the poor.

A year later, king Nebuchadnezzar was walking on the roof of his palace in Babylon enjoying his power and might when a voice from heaven proclaimed that he would be driven from human society, live with wild animals and eat grass for seven years. And so it came about that the great tyrant king lived like a wild animal and ate grass for seven

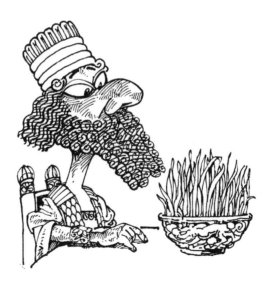

years, until, "I looked up at the sky, and my sanity returned."

Knowing what we do about the healing and rejuvenating properties of grass, it is likely that grass was at least partially responsible for the cure.

It took a war, millenia later, for wheatgrass to regain prominence as a healing agent when the grandmother of a young Ann Wigmore aided wounded soldiers in her native village in Lithuania, during the first world war. Grass was a traditional medicine used by many different healers of the 'old world'.

Ann Wigmore brought her grandmother's plant lore to the USA where she came to settle. During the years to follow, she subjected wheatgrass to extensive scientific testing. The result was that she was able to convince a large number of people of the value of wheatgrass for rebuilding health. The outcome of these studies shows wheatgrass to have spectacular medicinal properties.

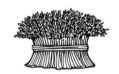

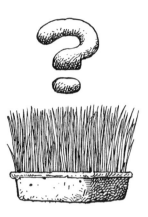

3

Wheatgrass – What is it?

Wheatgrass is sprouted wheat kernels which have been allowed to grow to the height of 6 inches or more, usually for 7 – 14 days (depending on warmth), either indoors or outdoors in trays or in the open ground. Wheatgrass is often grown in a special growing sheds with controlled lighting and other desired conditions. It can also be grown hydroponically without soil.

When the grass has reached its optimal level of growth, it can be juiced with a wheatgrass juicer or an ordinary blender. When a blender is used, liquify the wheatgrass with some pure water, with or without raw honey. It may also be chewed, frozen, dried or made into a tincture.

With proper planning and some basic equipment, most people can grow wheatgrass.

Fresh is best!

Enzymes in wheatgrass, which are very dynamic after seven days of growth, start rapidly breaking down after being juiced, so for best effects, drink wheatgrass juice immediately after juicing.

Wheatgrass juice will keep for about twelve hours in the refrigerator. Feed any left-overs to your animals and plants. Leftover juice can also be frozen in an ice-tray. Freezing does not destroy enzymes the way cooking does!

When is Wheatgrass at its most Nutritious?

Grass grown to the jointing stage (about a month) is at its most nutritious due to the fact that the root system has become more developed and better able to draw minerals and other essential nutrients from deep within the soil. Nutrient values of wheatgrass begin to decline at this point.

7 – day tray-grown wheatgrass (as seen in chapter 1) has incredible nutritional value, especially when it is grown in organic soil. Adding high quality kelp will help to mineralize the soil.

When wheatgrass is grown in trays, it has a shelf life of about 2 – 3 weeks, after which time it will start showing signs of wilting or shrinking. In its infancy wheatgrass

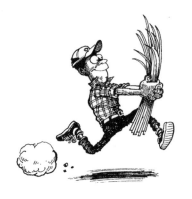

grows and develops very quickly; in a few days, its roots will cover the inside of the growing tray and are no longer able to draw sufficient nutrients from the soil. This is not the case when the kernels are planted out in an open field. Here the plant is given room to grow and develop. Some wheatgrass farmers combine the two techniques; planting the kernels in the open in selected areas and also growing it in trays. Growing wheatgrass in the open provides a backup if tray-grown wheatgrass fails to grow (this can happen if the kernels are old or they have been left to soak for too long).

7 – day old wheatgrass can also be mixed with older wheatgrass in order to provide an even more nutritious food.

How to grow Wheatgrass

You will need:

    16 standard seed trays with holes at the bottom
    1 lb. of whole-wheat kernels or Kamut, preferably organic
    2 large black refuse bags or plastic sheeting
    High quality organic compost
    2 thin boards, e.g. masonite,

approx. 24 inches x 36
inches each
Extra coverings such as canvas for
winter growing.

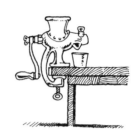

Sixteen trays of wheatgrass, grown once a week, will provide a family of four with super nutrition, by way of its juice and residue pulp (which is the by-product after juicing wheatgrass). Another by-product of wheatgrass is the mat, which helps to enrich the soil. See chapter 8 on how you can use the wheatgrass mat in your garden to benefit your plants. There will also be enough wheatgrass for family and friends in need of it and left-overs for cats, dogs and birds. Provided that you have all your equipment on site, planting the kernels, watering and covering them only takes about ten minutes. Wheatgrass is easy to grow and very rewarding.

Method

Place the kernels in a sieve and wash under running tap. Gently turn into a glass bowl and cover x 2 with puri-fied water. Cover the bowl and leave to soak for approx. 12 – 14 hours in summer and slightly longer in winter, about 16 hours. After this time, strain the seeds and soak water into a glass jug to make a ferment called Rejuvelac – see the following chapter.

Place the trays snugly together in a unit of four rows

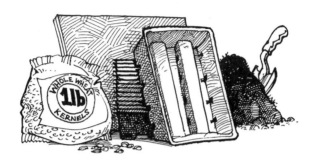

containing four seed trays. Half-fill the seed trays with
compost and place one handful of the soaked seeds onto
each tray. Spread the seeds out gently so that they just
touch, not overlap. Mist or spray gently. Cover the top of
the seed trays with the clean refuse bags or plastic sheeting.
Place boards on top of the plastic coverings. The black
refuse bags shut out the light. These conditions simulate
the action of the kernel within the soil (under ideal conditions). Germinating kernels, given water, warmth and
protection, will develop their own eco-culture; producing
burgeoning growth, especially within its root system.

If you plan to have your wheatgrass trays growing
outside, you may decide to place them on a specially
adapted table, i.e. a grid placed on a table frame will allow
excess water to drain off easily. The boards can be placed
on top of the plastic coverings for protection against the
sun in summer and the cold in winter. Canvas can be used
for added protection in winter.

Indoors, wheatgrass can be grown in trays and set in a

warm place such as a kitchen counter on top of newspaper (to absorb water residue). Follow the same procedure previously outlined concerning covering, watering, etc.

Mist or spray with a little water every day or two when the soil feels slightly dry. Keep the germinating kernels covered until the grass is about one or two inches high, a few days in summer, longer in winter. The grass grows very quickly at this stage and may grow more than one inch on a warm summer day. The emerging leaves are very pale yellow. Remove the plastic coverings and boards and place the trays in a protected, warm, light-shade spot. The grass is soon chlorophylated by the sun which fills the leaves with radiant, healing energy.

Water slightly for another 7 – 14 days (depending on whether it's summer or winter – wheatgrass takes longer in cold winter months). Your wheatgrass is now ready for harvest!

Avoid over-watering as this can cause mold or fungus growth. This disease may also attack young grasses when they are deprived of air for long periods. Remove coverings daily to allow circulation of air and keep coverings clean – they may get contaminated from bird droppings.

How much juice to take

As with any health regime, it is important to begin and proceed with caution.

Start off with an ⅛ tray (standard) of freshly juiced wheatgrass. This is about an ounce. Ideally, it is best to

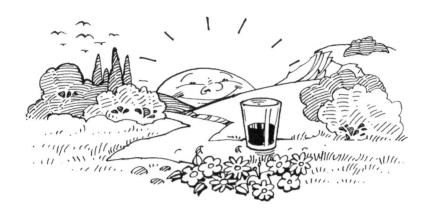

drink it first thing in the morning on an empty stomach. Wait for 20 minutes. It takes fast-acting Wheatgrass just 20 minutes to be assimilated into the system and to start its process of breaking down old mucous and toxins. Wheatgrass can be compared to a gentle detergent. Starting with the mouth, gums, teeth and then stomach, it filters into all the internal organs. It helps to purify the liver and aids the lymphatic system to carry away toxins from body cells. Some of these toxins may be many years old. Chances are that your body will be happy to let them go.

The bloodstream is where wheatgrass is particularly effective. Its cleansing nutrients purify and rebuild the blood. Wheatgrass may increase the production of hemoglobin and can help to reverse long-term diseases such as anemia and high blood pressure. According to Victoras Kulvinskas in *Survival into the 21st Century*, J. Hughes and A.L. Latner from the Department of Physiology, University of Liverpool, in a highly discriminative experiment, finally resolved the question of the blood regenerating capacity of chlorophyll. The following is a summary:

1. Pure chlorophyll in large doses has no effect on the speed of hemoglobin regeneration after hemorrhage. It seems that large doses are toxic to the bone marrow.

2. Very small doses of the pure chlorophyll markedly increase the speed of hemoglobin regeneration to approximately its previous level.

3. Crude chlorophyll is effective and non-toxic even in large doses.

4. Where effective, the anemic condition was overcome in 15 days.

Hughes concludes: "It seems therefore that the animal body is capable of converting chlorophyll to hemoglobin."

Wheatgrass contains crude chlorophyll and is described in number 3 above.

Growing your own versus taking Wheatgrass tablets and powders

Young wheatgrass shoots are extremely vital. Wheatgrass is a perfect, complete, whole food with enzymes, phytochemicals, vitamins and chlorophyll in perfect harmony to help create overall good health and help rid the body of toxins.

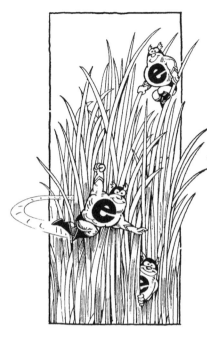

Wheatgrass Tablets and Powders

Wheatgrass contains abundant amounts of enzymes, and the conservation of these enzymes should be a primary consideration in the manufacture of wheatgrass tablets and powders. Manufacturers who use poor drying techniques will produce inferior products. According to Ann Wigmore in *The Wheatgrass Book*, "Enzymes are perhaps more important than any other active ingredient in wheatgrass. To date, literally hundreds of enzymes have been discovered in cereal grasses. An even more thorough study in the future may turn up thousands, because grass is a storehouse of enzymes."

Important factors which must be considered in the manufacture of Wheatgrass Tablets and Powders

1. Wheatgrass must be grown in nutritious live soil without the use of chemical pesticides, fertilizers or herbicides. Monitoring the soil is very important.
2. Oxidation may destroy certain nutrients within 30 minutes of harvesting, so speed is of the essence.

3. The grass must be washed in a non-toxic solution. Bleach can leave a toxic residue.

4. To ensure the continued activity of enzymes the extraction of the juice should be gentle so as to avoid crushing the cell walls. Certain freeze drying methods (lyophilization) avoid the heat applied to most wheatgrass tablets by the use of a gradual compression technique.

5. Immediate cooling of the juice and removal of oxygen by vacuum.

6. Ideally the juice is spray-dried at room temperature.

The above mentioned techniques for manufacturing wheatgrass tablets and powders are expensive and not all manufacturers heed these safeguards. Dr. Yoshihide Hagiwara spent over 30 years in the research and development of a naturally dried, nutritional supplement called Barleygreen. Through a special process of low temperature, he has been able to manufacture a product which ensures the survival of nutrients, and most importantly, of enzymes (1).

Good Reasons to Grow your Own

*Great Value: A 1 lb. packet of whole-wheat kernels or kamut will produce 16 trays of Wheatgrass and costs very little. Or buy communally in bulk for even better value.

*If you've got it, flaunt it! A carpet of wheatgrass looks good in the kitchen, bathroom and bedroom. It has the added advantage of oxygenating your living and sleeping areas.

*Good for a detox program: Besides the juice, used for drinking, the resulting leftover pulp can be used as a skin food. As much as 60% of this matter may be absorbed by the skin.

*Leave a tray out for dogs, cats and birds. They will love it!

*Nothing gets wasted. After harvesting the grass, the root mat can be used to either grow again, or placed roots up, it can be used in any area of the garden for re-building depleted soil.

Cost of Wheatgrass

1½ lb of wheat kernels will provide 64 standard trays of wheatgrass. Wheat kernels cost under $1 per pound, perhaps somewhat more for organic.

One tray (when approximately 6-7 days old) will serve four. 64 trays will provide super nutrition and alternative health therapy for 256 people.

Some Common Mistakes

* Purchasing old or infertile kernels. Purchase kernels at reputable health food stores to ensure freshness.
* Over watering.
* Leaving the trays covered for too long periods will cut off air which can cause mold or fungus. Even if

the germinating seeds do not need water, remove the plastic coverings daily for a few minutes in order to air the germinating seeds, before covering them up again.

* Plastic coverings can get contaminated with bird droppings. This can also cause mold and unfriendly bacteria.
* Young wheatgrass showing signs of wilting or drooping may be suffering from heat stroke or lack of water. Wheatgrass prefers light-shade conditions.
* Soaking the seeds for too long. Max about 16 hours.
* Making use of synthetic or depleted soil to grow your wheatgrass. If possible, make your own soil from organic compost.

Even if you do everything correctly, bear in mind that tray-grown wheatgrass has a shelf life of just a few weeks. This is due to the fact that when wheatgrass is grown in trays it soon reaches its maximum potential; it is very limited by its confinement in the tray, and the roots are soon starved of nutrients.

It Will Grow Again!

After harvesting your wheatgrass, its root-mat is ready for either the compost heap, where you can lay it down roots up, or for a protected spot in the garden where it can be replanted.

Start by pulling out the whole root-mass from the seed

tray (by tugging gently at one corner – it should all come out in one piece). If you are planting it out in the garden, water it everyday. Growing your own wheat to maturity is also very rewarding.

Drying the Pulp

Leave the pulp in the strainer until most of the juice has run out. Squeeze the pulp a little so that it is not too wet. Break off walnut sized rounds and flatten slightly. Place them onto paving stones or bricks in a sunny spot in the garden. Turn the pulp-rounds over every few hours in the course of the day. On a hot summers day they can dry out in about 8 hours. The drying process will attract ants and bees. Allow them to enjoy your harvest too.

Place these rounds in a paper bag. They will darken in time as they oxidize. Mold can result if the bag is tightly fastened – allow some opening for air to circulate. They can be added to bath mixtures – see chapter 7 on how to make Wheatgrass Bath-Milk and Bath Salts. The rounds contain a large amount of pro-vitamin A which converts to Vitamin A in the intestine. Vitamin A in this form is safe to use on the skin, and it is also protein-rich! Protein in wheatgrass is dramatically enhanced during the drying process. Raw honey, if used in the wheatgrass juice, will give your pulp added potency.

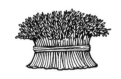

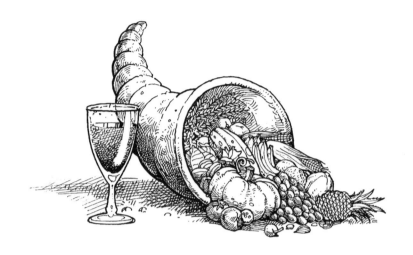

4

Longevity – Growing Young

A youthful skin, shining white teeth, boundless energy and a trim body belong to *everyone*.

Scientific research shows that plant substances can and do impact on our lives in many positive ways. On a physical level, we use these in the form of food or fluid as sustenance for our bodies. Used externally, plant substances can improve the condition of our hair, skin and nails.

On a subtle level, plant fragrances and essences work their special magic on the emotional and spiritual body. Fragrances can uplift us and transport us to memorable times in our past. Scent molecules move along the olfactory pathway to reach the innermost control centers of the brain – the place where fragrances "touch our hearts" (1).

Esoteric teachers have long believed that the brain's limbic system is where the body and soul connect. They also taught that healing takes place at this soul level.

Every illness has its cause and effect. Ideally, if there is any hope of a cure, causes need to be identified and understood. These are multifactorial, but a major cause of disease is the body's inability to access all of its nutrient intake.

Be Your own Healer

With a formidable body of knowledge available to us about juices, herbs and flowers, we can take stock of our lives and make changes that can not only make us feel better, but that can also make us look more youthful.

Wheatgrass has been extensively tested in the US for over 60 years. Much exciting information has come to light from this research, and we look here at those aspects that can free us from the normal bonds of aging.

According to researchers, the young wheat plant contains substances that can actually encourage cells to grow younger instead of older as the years go by (2).

There are many reasons why the body does not do this as a matter of course. One major factor of so-called "normal" wear and tear on the body is sun exposure, which causes premature wrinkling of the skin. There is nothing normal or predictable about looking old, especially when all the research shows that it is possible to look better, not older, with the passing of the years.

Other factors implicated in premature aging are stress and environmental pollution, both of which cause free-radical damage – chemical processes in the body shown to contribute to illness and disease.

It is true that we are what we eat. Some diets are not conducive to good health, and may lead to imbalances in the body. Just one example is an eating pattern that includes excessive intake of refined sugars and processed foods.

Yet with proper motivation, nutrition and moderate exercise, coupled with spiritual discipline and plant 'power', it is possible to create an environment in which the body can heal, and even rejuvenate itself.

Creating this environment is nothing short of an adventure!

Youth is characterized by boundless vitality and optimism. To enjoy this vital energy once more, even though decades may separate us from our youthful years, we need to cultivate it from within. The potential to do so is ever-present.

We first need to rid our systems of all those pollutants that drain us of our vital energy, because healing our bodies will assist in healing our minds and spirits. Stress may be physically and emotionally draining, but it can be rooted out of the body as effectively as toxins can be.

Fasting is an ancient, powerful and quick method of cleansing and rejuvenating the body. The down-side is that fasting can drain the body's reserves. However, there is a big difference between fasting and starving, and if you prepare the body correctly, a fast can give your health a powerful boost.

Before going on a fast, take at least a week to prepare your body by eating fresh fruit and vegetables and then drinking only vegetable and fruit juices.

How you break your fast is as important as how you prepare for it. If you overeat after a fast, you may undo all the good work from your voluntary abstinence from food. This is why fasting is best undertaken under a specialist's supervision.

If you want to eat your way to looking younger, then four to six moderate meals each day are the way to go. Small, frequent meals are ideal for increasing and maintaining stamina and mental vitality. Because wheatgrass juice is a complete food, it can be counted as a meal in itself.

Wheatgrass is also energizing and purifying to the system. During the process of chlorophyllation, wheatgrass absorbs light particles from the sun and stores these within its blades. This direct "sun-vitality" stimulates, purifies and rebuilds the system. It contains alkaline minerals that neutralize poisons, such as uric and other acids, that are released in the detoxification process. A radical change in diet should only be attempted under a specialist's direction.

Wheatgrass juice helps to create a more balanced internal environment. A rejuvenating program that incorporates wheatgrass and other 'live' food, in conjunction with exercise, has considerable beneficial effects.

Try an energizing alternative to fasting, and plan a 21-day, raw or semi-raw, rejuvenating health regime.

Checklist:

1. If you have the time, plant some basic greens that you may want to use. Sunflower, chickpeas and alfalfa sprouts grow easily indoors in a warm place. If you are using your own wheatgrass, plan your soaking and planting at least one week ahead of time for summertime use, and two to three weeks in winter. Or you can identify a high quality organic source.

2. Examine your body closely for areas that need regeneration. The skin is the largest organ in the body, and it may store toxins. Have a doctor check out any suspicious spots.

If you suffer from receding gums, wheatgrass pulp retained on diseased areas for 20 to 30 minutes a day helps to stimulate the growth of healthy tissue. For noticeable improvement, repeat this practice for a week or two. Four or five times a week thereafter will maintain the health of the gums. And your teeth will whiten in the process!

Fresh wheatgrass pulp is the path to radiant skin on the face and body. It will stimulate the skin, improve tone and texture, and remove blemishes. It is good for strengthening the capillaries in the skin. The pulp is also helpful to treat varicose veins. According to Ann Wigmore in *The Wheatgrass Book*, dried wheatgrass juice contains as much Vitamin A as carrots, kale, or apricots. Pro-vitamin A or carotene is converted in the intestines, as the need arises, into Vitamin A.

3. Write a synopsis of your goals, for example: weight loss (be realistic); building muscle mass; improving the condition of the teeth; improving texture and tone of the skin; improving general health, vitality and spiritual outlook.

4. A health rejuvenation plan needs back-up and support. If possible, work with others. This will lighten the load, and make the whole process much more fun.

5. On the morning of your first day, weigh yourself and record your weight.

6. Exercise is vital. If you have access to a gym, walk, cycle or row for 45 minutes to an hour three to four times per week.

7. Consider taking before and after photographs of yourself.

8. Check ingredients and buy organic foods and herbs whenever possible. Spices and herbs can be bought at health food shops.

Detoxification

The foods for this regime are carefully selected. Their main aim is to help maintain physical and mental energy. However, when there is a radical change in diet, with the use of strong cleansers such as wheatgrass juice, rejuvelac and herbs, you may experience the symptoms of detoxification. These may take the form, among others, of feelings of fatigue, changes in bowel movements or urinary action, and sweating. If you are concerned about any of these symptoms, consult a health practitioner to help you manage the detoxification more comfortably.

Balance

Balance in body, mind and spirit is a thread that runs through the intricate tapestries of most traditional healing systems.

The Greek physician, Hippocrates, who practiced the

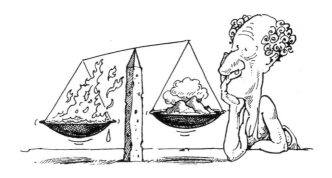

"Art of Healing" some 2,500 years ago, believed that the elements of earth, air, fire and water had to be balanced within the body for it to function properly.

Balance is also important in the ancient Indian traditional healing system of Ayurveda (life-knowledge or skill) and was practiced by the Brahmins from the earliest times. Air, sun and moon principles were seen to reflect the body in the form of air, fire and water. Balance was sought through the harmonious interplay between these three states.

Chinese traditional healing is premised on a balance between the complementary energies of yin (soft, feminine) and yang (hard, masculine).

Wheatgrass juice is a perfectly balanced whole-food. Its high chlorophyll content has strong, sun-vitality, which according to Chinese principles, is yang.

Being yang, chlorophyll has a strong fire quality that balances its moon or water element, which is yin. Its vitality stimulates and strengthens digestion and encourages the proper elimination of toxins. Chlorophyll's green pigment enriches the blood and increases the hemoglobin content. Mentally it helps promote a happy, harmonious disposition.

Restoring balance involves awareness of the body and correcting defective nutritional practices.

Is this regime right for you?

We are all different. Raw, cold food as suggested in the regime may not benefit all constitutions or suit all tastes. Warm, cooked food along with some raw plant foods may be more beneficial to those adversely disposed to raw foods. Be guided by your intuition.

Notes on Regime and Food

* *Fluids*

Water is the juice of the earth and represents 75% or more of our internal make-up. Clean, pure water has many health benefits, and its fluidity encourages the purification of our internal systems.

Drink at least six to eight cups of fluids daily, including mostly pure spring water or water that has been filtered. Herb teas may be sweetened with a little raw honey, sweet molasses, stevia or rice syrup.

Soy milk is a good source of calcium, and (obtainable from health shops) can be quickly made up in a blender by blending together 1 glass of purified water with 1 tablespoon of soya milk powder (or follow instructions on the label). Or you can buy it ready-made from health shops. Soy milk is very nourishing. Drink one or two glasses a day.

Tea

Pouring boiling water into a heated pot and adding

bags or herbs is a ritual that unites people from all over the world. It can also be a very healthy pastime.

Select tea according to your needs. Some herbs stimulate and others relax. Stress responds favourably to lemony balm or melissa , also known as bee-balm for its power to draw bees to its fragrant minty, lemony flowers at the end of summer.

The flowers and growing tips of lemon balm have great healing powers, especially for dispelling depression and anxiety. It can be used morning and night, and it helps to counteract insomnia. Lemon balm or melissa tea bags are available at health food stores.

Wash away your pains

For a relaxing and detoxifying bath, add 2 cups of mineral or Epsom salts to a jug with a lid. Pour into this mixture a little warm water and 4 to 5 drops each of pine and lavender aromatherapy oil. Shake well and pour into the hot bath. Agitate the water so that the salts and plant essences dissolve properly. Lie back and relax for 15 to 30 minutes.

Pine and lavender help to stimulate the circulatory system. A daily dose (or more) of wheatgrass juice will also improve the flow and quality of the blood.

Arthritis and rheumatism have many causes. Factors contributing to the diseases include old injuries, stress and poor diet. Most diets are too acidic, and a simple blood test will be able to show your acid/alkaline ratio. It should tend towards a pH of 7.4.

The skeletal system is not static. It has the ability to repair and rebuild itself in just a few months. Magnesium (richly supplied in wheatgrass) is able to "lock" calcium and other important minerals into bones and keep them there.

Calcium and magnesium requirements depend on your individual life-style. Conditions such as growth, pregnancy and stress require an adequate supply of these minerals. Current research suggests that the ratio between these minerals should be 1:1 or higher, in favour of magnesium.

Eating excessive amounts of bran can inhibit absorption of magnesium.

* *Cabbage*

Known as the "queen of crops", it has been used in successful rejuvenation regimes because of its cleansing and soothing effects on the internal and external system. When organically grown in high quality soil, it is high in minerals, including calcium and magnesium, that help to remineralize the body, and are easily assimilated.

Cabbage is also rich in folic acid. According to US studies, low levels of folic acid may contribute to heart disease.

The health benefits and digestibility of cabbage are greatest when it is eaten raw, as in cabbage juice, salad or sauerkraut. According to the Swiss "father" of natural healing, Dr. H. C. Vogel, raw cabbage juice (green or white cabbage) will improve and often cure such conditions as arthritis, stomach ulcers and metabolic disturbances (3).

* Fennel

In Italy it is known as "finocchio". All parts of this vegetable can be eaten; its bulb can be braised or roasted and its feathery new leaves and stalks are delicious in raw juices and in salads. The seeds make a good slimming tea. South African herb specialist and author Margaret Roberts advises not to exceed two cups per day for one week. Her method is: 1 cup chopped leaves and stalks boiled in 3 cups of water for 6-10 minutes (4).

Fennel is highly regarded by traditional health practitioners for its ability to dispel poisons from insects and other bites (it has antiseptic properties). It warms the stomach and helps ease colic and indigestion.

*Potato

The Scots affectionately call this wonderful vegetable a Tattie. When they are grown in rich organic soil, they are rich in Vitamin B6 and the minerals, phosphorus and potassium (also comparatively rich in copper). Raw potato juice is sometimes prescribed by a practitioner to do away with, or help neutralise, excessive stomach acid. In order to conserve their healing properties, cook very lightly or bake in their skins.

If you feel that you cannot face Cabbage Soup again, substitute this meal with an easy to prepare baked potato. Simply wash and scrub the potato, remove blemishes, and the 'eyes', prick all over with a fork and brush with a little oil. Bake in a moderate oven for approximately 35 – 45 minutes, depending on its size. Serve with a little cold-pressed olive oil.

Chickpea Sprouts

Chickpeas are protein-rich and make tasty sprouts. Wash chickpeas in a colander under a running tap. Place in a bowl, cover with purified water (x2) and allow to soak overnight. Place in a colander and cover. Rinse under a tap 1 – 2 times a day. They are ready to eat after 2 – 3 days.

* *Sunflower Sprouts*

Wash sunflower seeds (with hulls) and soak in purified water (x2) for about 8 hours. Strain into a large colander. Cover with a cloth and rinse 1 – 2 times a day for about 2 – 4 days. Remove hulls and keep in the refrigerator.

Alfalfa sprouts

Soak seeds in purifed water (x2) for about 8 hours and strain into a nylon colander. Cover with a cloth and rinse 1 – 2 times a day. They are ready in 3 – 5 days. Refrigerate for freshness.

Avocados

Very nourishing, it is best not to eat more than one-a-day of these delicious, enzyme-rich foods.

* *Almond*

This alkaline nut is a treasure-trove of important minerals, including: calcium, potassium, magnesium and phosphates. It also contains a high quality protein. For best digestibility, soak almonds overnight.

Pine nuts

Rich in protein and calcium, these nuts have a low carbohydrate content, so are good (in moderation) for weight watchers.

* *Rice*

Use unpolished brown rice which will assure a plentiful supply of important nutrients. Dr H.C.A. Vogel, In *The Nature Doctor*, says "Observations have shown that whole rice contains substances that keep the blood vessels elastic for much longer and it is for this reason that Asians seldom suffer from hardening of the arteries and high blood pressure". Sprouted rice can be obtained at specialty outlets.

Banana

Brimming with vitamin B6, folic acid and potassium, they will allay hunger pangs!

Mango

Enzyme-rich, this orange delight will sweeten your mood.

Papaya (pawpaw)

Papaya fruit has some extraordinary healing qualities, including the irradication of thread and other worms. It contains papain which is a predigestive agent and great for the digestion. Mashed-up papaya fruit can be applied to the skin to soften scar tissue.

Apple

'An apple a day' provides a wide range of vitamins and minerals. It also helps the digestion and can be given to children suffering from diarrhoea, in which case, liquify a well-washed apple (depipped) with a small amount of purified (or boiled) water. Allow the blended apple juice to brown before serving.

Pineapple

Pineapple contains, among many other nutrients, an enzyme called bromelain. Bromelain helps stimulate hormone secretion in the pancreas. Julie Stafford, author of *Juicing for Health*, Charles E. Tuttle Company Inc. 1994, says, "The bromelain enzyme has also been associated with the reduction of swelling and inflammation in rheumatoid arthritis, osteoarthritis and gout." Choose ripe, sweet-smelling ones.

Coconut milk

The coconut has cooling and soothing properties. The pure oil is a popular treatment for dry skin. In India it is used to massage babies.

Sesame seeds

Dr. H.C.A. Vogel, considers sesame seeds to be a perfect wholefood. Exceptionally rich in calcium, it also contains iron and phosphorus. This nutrient-rich food benefits children by supplying extra nourishment during the growing years. They strengthen the nerves and stimulate the heart muscle. Legend ascribes sesame with the power to

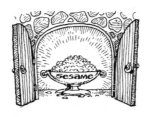

open doors, ie., 'Open Sesame!' Tahini is sesame seeds in pulp or butter form.

Kelp

Kelp, which is an 'ocean plant', is rich in minerals and trace elements. It also contains iodine. Dr. Vogel says, "If you suffer from Graves' disease (exophthalmic goitre) or hyperthyroidism, it is important to take kelp only in homoeopathic potency (1x-6x) because the effect of the remedy depends on the appropriate dilution being used."

* *Lemon*

The tangy juice of a lemon helps to alkalize acidity in the body. Use fresh to make your salad dressing.

* *Rejuvelac*

Try to start every day with ¼ glass of rejuvelac. Slightly acidic and not to everyone's taste, this is a mildly fermented drink made from wheat kernels. It has the strongest effect when taken by itself but it can also be mixed with cold fruit juice to make it more palatable.

Rejuvelac is a tonic that greatly enhances digestion and peristalsis. It is thus helpful in conditions such as constipation. It is rich in lactobacilli, phosphates, enzymes and aspergillus oryzae. Amylases, which are produced from aspergillus oryzae, assist in the break-down of large molecules of starch, glucose and glycogens (5). Vitamins B, C and E are also supplied, as are proteins.

The flavor of fresh rejuvelac is lemony. Do not drink it if it tastes putrid. Unlike wheatgrass, which has an alkalizing effect on the body, rejuvelac is moderately acidic and is not suitable for everyone.

If you do not wish to use rejuvelac, squeeze half a lemon into ½ glass of water.

A 20 – 30 minute wait is ideal for digestion to take place. Follow with 1 oz. of wheatgrass juice (1 oz. or less up to 2 or 3 times a day if tolerated). It takes fast-acting wheatgrass juice just 20 minutes to start its detoxification process.

As the wheatgrass juice breaks down toxins, you may feel some discomfort. Lie down for a little while and do some zone therapy (6). This can be done by gently, yet firmly. manipulating the effected area to allow the body to expel gasses, which may be the cause of the trouble.

If your reaction is uncomfortably strong, you may decide to halve your wheatgrass dose next time around.

Try and keep up the practice of drinking rejuvelac (or lemon) and wheatgrass juice every morning. Take half the dose if 1 oz. is too difficult.   Drink another 1 oz. dose (or less) 20 minutes before lunch and supper.

Over 50's

Losing large amounts of weight after the age of 50 years of age can be a stress on the body and be counterproductive. A gentle approach is indicated.

Wheatgrass is rich in magnesium. The daily requirement of this important mineral is around 400 – 800 mg. Wheatgrass and rejuvelac help the system to metabolize more efficiently.

No matter what your age, exercise remains an important factor in optimum well-being. Regular walks, swimming and cycling promote the health of the skeletal structure.

Indulge in calcium-rich snacks, cold-pressed oils, sweet molasses and raw honey.

* *Take time to smell the roses.*

Smell has been described as the most mystical of all our senses. The personality of the plant is said to be in the flower. It is the most dynamic part and has the ability to uplift the spirit.

The 21-day Wheatgrass Rejuvenation plan

This plan makes it possible to navigate the day according to principles of energy needs and digestion. Digestion functions best when fewer foods are eaten at the same time. Greens consumed with either proteins or starches/carbohydrates in a meal, have added benefits.

If you cannot do without your daily bread, try to

obtain the best quality stone-ground, brown bread and lightly toast it. Or even better, prepare your own sprouted bread!

Millet is an alkaline grain loaded with important minerals including silica, and is very nourishing. It is easily obtained at health food shops and can be used to make a variety of healthy dishes.

Recipes used in the 21-day Wheatgrass Rejuvenation plan can be found in chapter 5.

The 21 day Wheatgrass Rejuvination plan can be broken down into three phases:

1. Days 1 to 10: Eating and drinking become progressively more raw.
2. 1 raw day.
3. Days 12 to 21: Re-orientation towards a semi-raw diet.

Day 1

On arising: Drink a quarter glass of rejuvelac or half a lemon squeezed into half a glass of water. Sweeten with a little raw honey, stevia or rice syrup if necessary. Wait 20 minutes (or longer) for digestion to take place, and then drink wheatgrass according to your capabilities.

1-3 oz. per day can usually be tolerated to begin with.
1 9" by 6" tray of wheatgrass will produce between 5 and 8 oz. of wheatgrass juice.

1 oz. is roughly ⅛ of a tray or a small bunch.

If you are buying your wheatgrass from a supplier, check their recommendations. Wheatgrass can be juiced in a wheatgrass juicer and drunk by itself or as a blended juice. See chapter 5.

Breakfast : Fruit or vegetable juice.

For optimum digestibility, choose fruits that harmonize with each other. Tropical fruits such as mango, pineapple and paw-paw or apples and pears blend well. Digestibility is enhanced when a single fruit is used exclusively, hence the term "mono-fruit" meals.

Some fruits prefer to be eaten alone:

*Melon helps to relieve water retention. Choose one of the many varieties.

*Grapes are a high-energy fruit which contain cleansing and revitalizing substances. They have been used successfully to fight cancer.

Rejuvelac, wheatgrass and most fruits take about 20 to 30 minutes to digest. A carbohydrate meal can take 3 hours or more.

Snacks : (Eat on an empty stomach)

Many people depend on pasteurized milk and other dairy products to supply the body's calcium and magnesium needs. A variety of plant sources including wheatgrass, cabbage, sesame seeds and soybeans can supply an excellent quality calcium that is easily absorbed by the body. These make tasty snacks!

Tahini, a paste made from pounded sesame seeds, is also a good source of calcium. See Tahini Dips in the following chapter.

Lunch and supper: Cabbage soup.

Day 2

On arising: Repeat Day 1. Half a glass of Rejuvelac followed 20 minutes later by wheatgrass juice. Drink according to your capability. If 1 oz. is too difficult, try halving the dose. Allow 20 minutes for the wheatgrass juice to digest before eating breakfast.

Breakfast: Fruit or vegetable juice.

Lunch and supper: 1 oz. or less of wheatgrass juice may be drunk 20 minutes before eating. Cabbage soup or Chili Chickpeas.

Day 3

On arising: Repeat Day 1. Half a glass of rejuvelac followed 20 minutes later by 1 oz. wheatgrass juice. Wait 20 minutes before eating.

Breakfast: Mono-fruit or Almond Vanilla.

Lunch and supper: Cabbage Soup or Braised fennel.

1 oz. or less of wheatgrass juice may be drunk 20 minutes before eating.

Day 4

On arising: Repeat Day 1. Half a glass of rejuvelac followed 20 minutes later by 1 oz., or less of wheatgrass juice. Allow 20 minutes digestion time before breakfast.
Breakfast: Mono-fruit such as 1 or 2 sweet grapefruits.
Lunch and supper: Cabbage or Purple-heart salad.
Drink 1 oz. or less of wheatgrass juice 20 minutes before.

Day 5

On arising: Repeat Day 1.
Breakfast: Sunshine Smoothy.
Lunch and supper: Cabbage Salad or Sprouted Pineapple Rice.

Day 6

On arising: Repeat Day 1.
Breakfast: Fruit Soup.
Lunch and supper: Cabbage Soup or Sunflower and alfalfa salad.

Day 7

On arising: Repeat Day 1.
Breakfast: Sesame and sunflower milk.
Lunch and supper: Sprouted Pineapple Rice or Tropical Fruit Salad.

Day 8

On arising: Repeat Day 1.
Breakfast: Coconut Milk or Tropical Fruit Salad.
Lunch and supper: Cabbage Soup or Sauerkraut.

Day 9

On arising: Repeat Day 1.
Breakfast: Mono-fruit.
Lunch and supper: Cabbage Soup or Curried Flowers.

Day 10

On arising: Repeat Day 1.
Breakfast: Mono-fruit.
Lunch and supper: Cabbage Soup or Almond Apple Pie.

Day 11 (All raw)

On arising: Repeat Day 1.
Breakfast: Mono-fruit.
Lunch and supper: Salads or raw vegetables. If this is too strenuous, have Cabbage Soup.

Days 12 to 21

Go backwards from Day 11. Repeat days 10, 9, 8, 7, 6, 5, 4, 3, 2 and 1. You have completed 21 days! Even if all you did was drink wheatgrass every day, and adhered to some food-combination principles, you will be looking and feeling greatly improved.

The following testimonials are from people who have used wheatgrass to improve aspects of their health.

Here is a testimonial from Taryn Lockhart, after her 21-Day Wheatgrass Diet:

"I am happy to say that since I went on the 21-day Wheatgrass diet, my outlook on life has changed. Not only did the program give me more vitality, but it changed my attitude generally, because I started feeling great. I have also lost 13 lbs. in total, and I didn't even intend to lose weight.

I am slimmer now and I feel that my body has rejuvenated itself and that I'm a new person living in a different body. I must admit that I didn't stick to the diet 100%, but the 90% did the world of good for me and the way my body feels."

"Hi Li,

First, I have to thank you for your continuous supply of this wonderful stuff, wheatgrass. Every morning I make this juice, where I mix it with some raw fruits and carrots, lemon and honey and it tastes delicious. With the pulp of the wheatgrass I rub my face and hands, and the liver or age marks in my face have about disappeared. Tai swears that it is the wheat grass pulp, which stopped the bleeding gum condition he has had, off and on for as long as he can remember. It has also whitened some discoloration on his teeth.

Tai, my husband, Demian, my son, and I have been taking wheatgrass for about 5 years. We are feeling very healthy and would hate to ever miss it.

Love,
Agna Smirnoff Krige, Jhb."

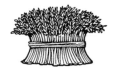

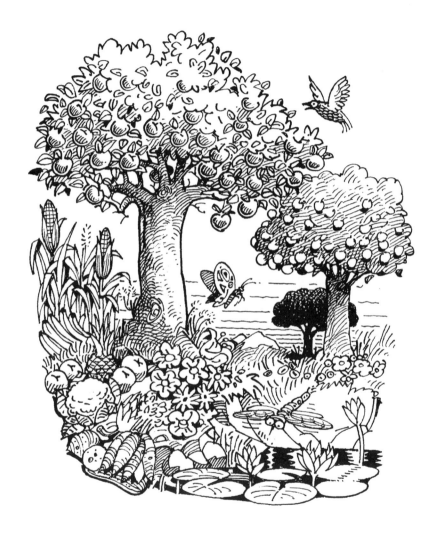

5

Become a Green Gourmand!

Picture a beautiful orchard. Abundant fruit and berries cascade down from lush verdant branches. The sun trickles through and warms the plants and flowers growing underneath. Vegetables lean up against wheat and barley grasses for protection, and a rich, strong fragrance draws the dragonfly to the water's edge. Bees, birds and butterflies live in harmony.

The foods we eat need to come from such a happy environment, to produce a harmonious mix of nutrients so important for the proper rejuvenation of the body. Plants lovingly grown, in optimal organic soil, cannot fail but to give us the balance and vitality so important in the busy lives we lead.

As we move into a new millennium, it becomes increasingly clear that if we all work together, no one will have to go hungry! It has been estimated that if just 10% of the world population were to move from consumption to production, even just raising our own gardens, there would be enough food for all (1).

Recipes in this chapter benefit from the use of fresh produce. So respond to the call of nature, and grow your own wherever and whenever possible.

The Ferment

Fermentation is a chemical reaction in which an organic molecule splits into simpler substances (2).

In *rejuvelac*, which is the soured soak water of washed wheat kernels, this fermentation produces natural enzymes and lactic acid. Of lactic acid, Dr. Kuhl, a German researcher, says "Lactic acid destroys harmful intestinal bacteria and contributes to the better digestion and assimilation of nutrients. Fermented foods can be considered predigested foods. They are easily metabolized, even by persons with weak digestive organs. Fermented foods cleanse the intestinal tract and provide a proper environment for the body's own vitamin productions within the intestine. They also help a person with constipation problems."

Rejuvelac

1 lb. whole wheat kernels or kamut, preferably organic
2 pints purified water
1 square of paper towelling
1 glass jug

Use wheat which is indigenous to your environment. In America the hard, red, winter wheat-kernels are superior for germination and growth.

Pour the wheat kernels into a strainer and wash thoroughly under the tap. Place in a jug and cover with water. Remove any loose stalks and other debris. Cover and leave for approximately 12 – 14 hours in summer or 14 – 16 hours in winter.

Strain and return the soak water into the glass jug. Gently wet the square of paper towelling and cover the mouth of the jug with it. Press all the way around the sides. It will dry tautly and prevent any foreign material from entering the Rejuvelac. The soak water needs a temperature of between 68 and 100 degrees 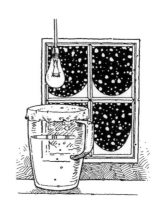 Farenheit to ferment. Light is necessary for the fermentation process to occure, so place your jug on a warm kitchen window sill. In cold conditions, you may need to devise a system using light bulbs or other warming devices (3).

Leave undisturbed for 2-3 days. This is when the ferment is at its most nutritious. Covered and refrigerated, it should keep for weeks. Use a little of your old rejuvelac to activate a new batch. The taste should be slightly sour with a lemonish flavour. Do not consume if it tastes foul. If in any doubt, compost it.

Rejuvelac is delicious mixed with fruit juice. It can also be used to make seed yogurt or cheeses. The soaked wheat kernel can be sprouted and made into sprout bread. Or simply plant it – either outdoors in the open or in trays. See chapter 3 for how to grow wheatgrass.

Sprout Bread or Essene Bread

4 cups wheat kernels or kamut
4 cups rejuvelac or purified water
Warm sun

Wash the kernels in a large plastic or nylon strainer under the tap and soak for 12 – 16 hours in purified water. Run the kernels back through the strainer and keep the soak water. This liquid can be placed covered on a warm window sill and left to sour slightly.

The soaked kernels, now in the strainer, can be left covered with a cloth for another day or two. Rinse with a little purified water once or twice during the course of the day. If you use Rejuvelac to make your bread instead of water, it will have a stronger, slightly sour taste. It will, however, be enriched with protein, phosphates, lactobacilli and asperigillus oryzae from which amylases are a derivative. Great for digestion and for rebuilding the intestinal flora! It also contains large amounts of B vitamins. Sour dough bread has a milder flavour compared to Sprout Bread or Essene Bread. Sour dough is made by allowing flour and water to ferment (often in a

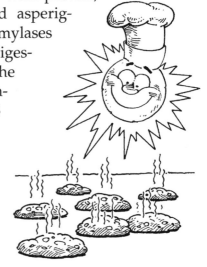

special machine) which in turn produces natural yeasts and an abundance of gasseous molecules to aid in the raising of the dough.

Method

Half-fill the blender with rejuvelac or purified water. Start off by adding half a cup of sprouted wheat kernels – one or two day old sprouts. Blend well and gradually add more. As the blender fills up, pour the wheat sprout mix into the strainer (with a bowl underneath) and pound this pulp so that as much liquid as possible comes through. Return this liquid into the blender and carry on blending until all the sprouts have been added. You may need to add more Rejuvelac. Strain further, to produce a consistency which will hold together. Press into thin wafers approximately 2 inch in diameter and set them out to "cook" in the sun. Place on oiled paper or straight onto bricks, preferably on a wall or table, to keep the ants and bugs off. Turn the wafers every few hours until they are dry on the outside and slightly moist inside.

These breads make a good complement to salads or soup. They can also be made into pizza or served with a dip. For sweet sprout bread, add raw honey and cinnamon to taste while blending.

Curds and Whey

Rejuvelac can also be used to make soy cheese or yogurt. Below I describe the process of making curds and whey from sprouted soy beans. Whey is the liquid that separates from the solids during a dynamic process or change of state. This process is similar to the making of cheese from clotted milk. Here the watery liquid separates from the curd when the milk is clotted.

Soy Cream Cheese

½ lb. of soy beans, preferably organic – obtainable from health food stores
3 cups rejuvelac – see recipe for making rejuvelac
Glass jar

Soak soybeans for 24 hours and leave covered in a large strainer for a further 16 hours. Rinse every 4 – 6 hours. (This water can be left, covered, on a warm window sill for 1 – 2 days for a strong-tasting soy rejuvelac).

Place the rejuvelac into a blender and add 1 cup of sprouted soy beans. Blend well. Gradually add the remaining sprouted soy beans. If the blender fills up too much, pour everything into a strainer and collect the liquid in a bowl. Pour the strained soy sprout liquid back into the blender and proceed by adding further soy sprouts and rejuvelac until it is all used up.

Strain ingredients into the glass jar. Grind the pulp against the strainer in order to extract as much of the pulp as possible. Stir the mixture – it should have the consistency of frothy cream. Cover the top of the mouth of the jar with a damp paper towel and leave in a warm place, undisturbed, for 4 – 6 hours.

Pour into a large strainer on top of a bowl and refrigerate for about an hour. The whey will separate from the curd, which is a soft mass, and seep into the bowl. It is very nutritious and can be mixed back into the curd if you want to make a soy yogurt.

Wheatgrass Juice Makes Tasty, Refreshing Drinks

A harmonious mix of herbs, flowers and honey can convert wheatgrass into the *champagne* of raw food drinks. For this you need a blender. If you feel more comfortable using a wheatgrass juicer (less oxidation), you can add the resultant juice to your blended and strained flower, herb and honey concoction.

Brain-Boosting Wheatgrass Nectar

1 tray wheatgrass, cut down to the roots and washed
1 tablespoon raw honey
Edible flowers and herbs that you may have available:
6 – 8 rosemary flowers
4 – 6 pineapple sage blooms
4 gotu kola leaves
6 – 8 marjoram flowers
6 – 8 basil flowers
6 – 8 alfalfa flowers (lucerne)

2 – 3 sprigs peppermint
2 – 3 sprigs thyme
1 catmint flower head
1 chunk ginger, peeled and chopped
2 pints cold water

Blend together all the above ingredients (except for the red pineapple sage blooms) and strain into a glass jug. Chop sage flowers and sprinkle on top for decoration. Due to the oxidation process blended wheatgrass will produce a frothy green 'head'. It is safe to drink.

Visualization Juice

1 tray wheatgrass, cut down to the roots and washed
1 tablespoon raw honey
Any of the following herbs and flowers:
6 – 8 rosemary flowers
1 flower head of yarrow
2 sprigs of peppermint or mint
4 red clover flowers
2 nasturtium flowers
2 – 3 clary sage flowers
6 – 8 small blossoms of lemon balm or 1 inch piece of growing tip
6 – 8 lavender flowers or 1 inch piece of growing tip
½ inch piece of red chilli pepper
1 teaspoon non-irradiated cinnamon – obtainable at health food stores

½ of a lemon, squeezed

2 pints cold water

Blend together all the ingredients and strain into a glass jug. Serve immediately.

Note: Never use clary sage if you are suffering from epilepsy as this potent herb effects the nervous system. Do not use in conjuction with medication containing iron.

Wheatgrass Ginger Ice-Cubes

Small handful of wheatgrass, cut down to the roots and washed

2½ Cups purified water

1 – 3 inch piece of ginger, peeled and chopped

Strainer

Standard Ice-Tray

Pour the water into the blender. Add wheatgrass and ginger. Blend for a few minutes and strain into the ice-tray. Place in the freezer section of the refrigerator. It should keep for a month or more. Use in soups, salads, sauces and sweets.

This recipe can also be used to make Chili Ice-Cubes. Substitute 1 – 2 red chilies for the ginger. Very hot!

Wheatgrass – Rejuvenation Plan

The following recipes are mentioned in the preceding chapter. They serve 2.

Tahini Dips

Sweet Tahini – Mix 1 tablespoon or more of tahini with 1 tablespoon of sweet molasses. 1 or more tablespoons of raw honey may be added. Serve with chilled pieces of fruit such as peeled and sliced mango or papaya (pawpaw).

Savory Tahini – Spread 1 or 2 teaspoons tahini paste on a few clean young celery stalks (leaves removed). Season with Braggs Amino's and fresh lemon juice.

Cabbage Soup

1 cabbage, washed and chopped
2 red peppers, thinly sliced
small bunch chives, washed and sliced
1 – 2 cloves garlic, peeled and crushed
1 tablespoon high quality kelp powder
1 leaf each of sage and bay
a small handful of parsley and thyme
a handful of sunflower and alfalfa sprouts
½ teaspoon each of marjoram, celery, fennel and rosemary flowers, washed and chopped (when available) or 1 – 2 nasturtium flowers
1 – 2 tablespoons of cold pressed olive oil
a squeeze of lemon
4 cups boiling water
Braggs Amino's to taste (optional)

Heat the oil and stir-fry the peppers for 1 – 2 minutes. Add cabbage and stir quickly for another few minutes.

Add boiling water, stir in bay leaf, sage, parsley and thyme and switch off heat. Cover the pan with a tightly fitting lid and leave for about 5 minutes to cool down slightly. Stir in crushed garlic, kelp powder and lemon juice. Season to taste. Garnish with sunflower and alfalfa sprouts, chopped chives and flowers. Frying with olive oil causes it to oxidize which is not suitable for those suffering from high cholestrol.

Hot Raw Chili Chickpeas

4 cups sprouted chickpeas
1 red pepper, washed and thinly sliced
1 small cabbage, washed and shredded
small bunch parsley, washed and chopped

Sauce – In a blender, blend together:
1 tablespoon lemon juice
1 tablespoon honey
1 inch chunk ginger, peeled and cut finely
1 tablespoon sesame oil
2 tablespoons soy oil
1 cup hot water
1 chili ice-cube (see recipe), or cayenne pepper to taste

Steam cabbage for a few minutes and place into a heated dish. Top with chickpeas and pour the sauce over. Garnish with red pepper and parsley.

Almond Vanilla

Night before – soak 1 cup of almonds in 2 cups of purified water. In a liquidizer blend together the soaked almonds and water in conjunction with 1 tablespoon of raw honey (optional) and a dash of vanilla essence (obtainable at health shop). Add extra cold water if need be. Strain or drink 'au naturale'.

Fennel Mayonnaise

Night before – soak 1 cup of pine nuts in 2 cups of purified water. If pine nuts are unavailable, use almonds or sunflower seeds.

2 large fennel bulbs (stalks removed) cut down the middle and washed
1 tablespoon cold-pressed olive oil
½ cup boiling water

Mayonnaise – mix together:

1 tablespoon tahini
1 – 2 teaspoons sweet molasses (optional)
1 garlic, crushed
Small bunch parsley and chives, washed and finely chopped
fresh lemon juice to taste

Braise the fennel for 5 minutes in a frying pan, first in the oil for a few minutes and then add the boiling water. Cover with a tightly fitting lid and turn off the heat. Allow fennel to cool down for about 5 minutes. Pour the vegetable into a heated dish. Spread with mayonnaise and top with chopped pine nuts.

Purple Heart Salad

4 large carrots, scrubbed and finely grated
½ onion, finely chopped
1 lemon, squeezed
1 teaspoon kelp or sea salt
1 handful of sunflower sprouts, washed
1 handful of alfalfa sprouts

In a salad dish mix together the first four ingredients. Refrigerate for 15 minutes. Decorate with sunflower and alfalfa sprouts and serve.

Sunshine Smoothy

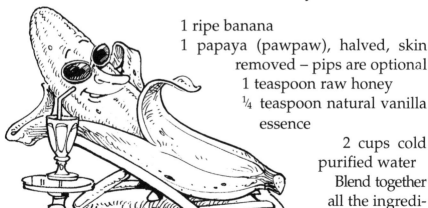

1 ripe banana
1 papaya (pawpaw), halved, skin removed – pips are optional
1 teaspoon raw honey
¼ teaspoon natural vanilla essence
2 cups cold purified water

Blend together all the ingredients in a

liquidizer and serve immediately.

Fruit Soup

3 – 4 ripe avocados, peeled and mashed
3 – 4 ripe tomatoes, washed
1 cup raw beet juice
2 – 3 cups cold purified water (according to desired consistancy)
dash lemon
kelp or sea salt (very little) to taste
1 handful of basil and marjoram flowers (if available)
In a liquidizer, blend together the water, beetjuice and tomatoes for 1 – 2 seconds. Pour the liquid into a soup turine, mix in the mashed avocado, season and garnish with flowers.

Avocado Sprout Salad

½ onion, finely chopped
4 tablespoons cold-pressed olive oil (flax or hemp oil may be used instead)
1 lemon, squeezed
kelp or sea salt to taste
2 – 3 ripe avocados, peeled and sliced
2 cups each of sunflower and alfalfa sprouts
Mix together the first 4 ingredients. Place the avocado into a salad dish and pour the dressing over, mixing in gently. Incorporate the sprouts and serve immediately.

Sesame and Sunflower Milk

½ cup sunflower seeds
¼ cup sesame seeds
Raw honey to taste
3 cups purified water
Soak seeds overnight in the water. In a liquidizer blend together the soaked seeds and water, with honey to taste. Strain and serve immediately.

Sprouted Pineapple Rice

1 pineapple, husk removed and juiced
1 tablespoon sesame oil, cold-pressed
½ onion, peeled and finely chopped
½ lemon, juice
kelp or sea salt to taste
2 – 3 cups sprouted rice
a pinch of rosemary or other edible flowers
Mix together the first 5 ingredients. Check seasoning. Mix in the sprouted rice and decorate with flowers.

Tropical Fruit Salad

1 papaya (paw-paw), halve, remove pips and skin – cut up small
1 ripe mango – peel off the skin and cut into small cubes
1 – 2 ripe bananas, sliced

1 ripe, sweet pineapple, juiced – or 1 orange, squeezed
A few flowers in season: lime, orange, scented geranium, chopped fine
Mix together all the ingredients and top with chopped flowers. Chill in the refrigerator for 10 – 15 minutes before serving.

Sauerkraut

(This recipe can be doubled or tripled)

1 large cabbage, wash and retain some whole leaves to cover
2 teaspoons kelp
1 teaspoon fresh or dried dill
2 – 3 ground juniper berries

Grate the cabbage. Half fill a bowl and pound until it becomes juicy. Place clean cabbage leaves over. On top of the leaves place something heavy in order to press down on the cabbage. Cover with a towel and set in a warm place. Leave undisturbed for about a week. Remove weight and discard outer leaves. Some residue may have formed on the top layers, this can be removed. Place in a glass jar with a tightly fitting lid. The sauerkraut will keep in the refrigerator for about one month. This recipe is adapted from Ann Wigmore's *Hippocrates Diet*.

Curried Flowers

3 potatoes, washed and chopped up small

1 inch piece of ginger, peeled and chopped finely
1 clove garlic, crushed
1 teaspoon cayenne pepper
1 teaspoon each of coriander and cumin
3 carrots, juiced – retain the pulp
seasoning, sea salt or kelp
2 – 3 cups boiling water
½ a lemon, squeezed
small handful of alfalfa or coriander flowers, chopped
fine (if available)

Heat the oil and fry the ginger for a few minutes. Pour the boiling water over and add the potatoes. Boil until just tender. Switch off the heat and allow to cool for about 5 – 10 minutes. Add the carrot juice and pulp, lemon, coriander, cumin, garlic and seasoning. Stir in flowers.

Almond Apple Pie

2 cups almonds (soaked overnight)
1 tablespoon maple syrup
Filling:
5 – 6 slightly stewed apples sweetened with stevia
1 teaspoon cinnamon

In a processer, process soaked almonds until fine. Incorporate maple syrup until the mixture holds together. Press into a serving dish and fill with the stewed apples. Sprinkle with cinnamon.

Vibrant Vegetable Juices – Drink your health!

Nutritious drinks made from fresh vegetables and combined with wheatgrass will assist the body in detoxifying, remineralizing and rebuilding.

Brimming with natural enzymes, chlorophyll, aminoacids, vitamins, minerals and lecithin, wheatgrass is the perfect, complete whole-food. It will compensate for nutritional deficiencies and add vigor to your step. Combine wheatgrass with vegetables for even more impact!

For optimal health and nutrition use organically grown vegetables wherever possible.

Organic farming is a system that is environmentally friendly and free of chemicals. Freshly harvested organic crops may not look as good as those "forced" to grow with fertilizers, but they always outshine their chemically raised cousins in taste and health value.

Healthy Vegetables

1. Carrots

They are loaded with betacarotene, vitamins B1, B2 and B6, as well as vitamins C and K. Minerals include rich amounts of phosphorus, potassium, iron and calcium. Copper, zinc, potassium, magnesium and cobalt are also supplied. The carotene that gives carrots their orangey color influences the production of sex hormones and improves the function of the sex glands (1).

The mega-nutrients contained in carrots help to boost brain function (including memory), and enhance the health of the eyes, teeth and skin.

This vegetable also helps to boost the immune system and detoxify the liver.

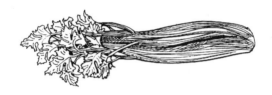

2. Celery

The roots, stalks and leaves, used on a regular basis, assist in preventing stones or renal gravel (2). This alkaline food-medicine is useful for the treatment of arthritis, rheumatism and gout, and helps to eliminate excess uric acid. It also helps to normalize blood sugar levels.

3. Cabbage

This vegetable contains high concentrations of organic chlorine and sulphur that aid in cleansing mucus membranes of the stomach and intestinal tract (3). Ulcers respond well to raw cabbage juice.

4. Beetroot

Betalaine, responsible for the red colour of the juice, stimulates the function of the liver cells and bile ducts.

There is anecdotal evidence of beetroot's anti-tumor activity: In an article entitled "Organic Beet Juice strengthens the immune system" (4), Dr. John Heinerman recounts how Dr. Alexander Ferenczi, at the hospital in Csoma in Hungary, treated cancer patients between 1955 and 1959 with organic beetroot (juiced and grated). Twenty one of the 22 patients who followed the therapy "experienced varying degrees of improvement as demonstrated by shrinking their tumors, noticeable weight gains, decreased ESR, and definite improvements in appetite and general health".

Beetroot is also a very good source of iron that can help to improve the red blood corpuscles. Dr. H.C.A. Vogel advises that you give a "pale" child a small glass of beetroot juice before meals every day, morning and evenings (5).

5. Cucumber

Apart from its cooling and astringent properties, this vegetable has excellent diuretic properties. It contains 0.2-0.1 gm. percent magnesium.

6. Red Pepper

This vegetable contains up to nine times as much betacarotene and twice as much vitamin C as green peppers (6). It also contains vitamins B1, B2, C and E. Handle them with care as they contain capsicin that can irritate the skin and mucus membranes. Too much red pepper can cause gastritis.

7. Tomato

Sun-ripened, they contain many vitamins, including large amounts of betacarotene, vitamins C and E, and the mineral potassium. Lycopene, a carotenoid-antioxidant, helps to reduce the risk of cancers (prostate cancer and cancers of the gastrointestinal tract). Pink grapefruit, watermelon, guavas and apricots are other lycopene-rich foods (7).

8. Ginger

This spicy root is a good energizer. Its warming properties make it a good remedy for colds and flu. It also helps to stimulate the circulation, aids fluid retention, and relieves nausea and travel sickness.

9. Fennel

This delicious vegetable is rich in calcium and magnesium, and has remarkable healing and soothing properties.

10. Garlic

An immune booster with antiseptic, antiviral and antibacterial properties, it is also used successfully for the treatment of high blood pressure. Other high-blood-pressure "fighters" are yarrow, hawthorn, dandelion and wheatgrass.

Garlic is said to be useful to eliminate build-up of fatty deposits in the arteries.

Use in small amounts only.

11. Other beneficial greens

Small amounts of dandelion greens, mustard greens,

watercress, broccoli and small amounts of herbs, flowers and sprouts can also be juiced for good health. Do not ever use any herb or flower that you are not sure of.

Soaking seeds in water and allowing them to grow awakens the vital energy of the plant. This "power-burst" provides us with a nutritious, easy-to-digest food that is light on the taste buds, and is virtually calorie-free.

Fresh vegetable juices are also delicious! They furnish the body with essential micronutrients, supply energy and boost the immune system.

A juicer is necessary to make the following recipes.

Magnesium 'A' Juice

½ green or red pepper (capsicum), washed and chopped, with seeds removed
1 small bunch spinach, washed and chopped
2 parsnips, washed and scrubbed
2 beetroots, washed and scrubbed, including tops
½ teaspoon kelp
Fresh lemon juice
Juice the first four ingredients, stir in the kelp and lemon juice to taste.

Slim Jim

6 young stalks of celery with foliage – washed, scrubbed and chopped
1 chopped cucumber

1 – 2 stalks fennel including foliage, washed and scrubbed
2 tomatoes, washed and cut up
1 sprig young lucerne, or a handful of alfalfa sprouts
½ inch piece of ginger, peeled and cut up
½ teaspoon kelp
juice of ½ a lemon
Juice all the ingredients. Stir in kelp and lemon juice to taste.

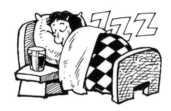

Slumber Juice

6 young carrots with tops, well-washed
1 small lettuce, washed
2 lemon balm leaves, washed
¼ inch sprig of lavender leaves or flowers
1 teaspoon raw honey, dissolved in a small amount of hot water
Juice the first four ingredients. Stir in honey water.

Titan's Tonic

6 young carrots with foliage, well-washed
1 or 2 healthy young radishes, including foliage, well-washed
½ small red pepper (capsicum) washed, with seeds removed and chopped
1 beetroot including tops, washed, scrubbed and chopped
2 or 3 leaves of young cabbage, washed and cut up
1 tablespoon alfalfa sprouts
1 gotu kola leaf, washed (optional)
Small sprigs of oregano, thyme and basil, washed
Juice of ½ a lemon
¼ teaspoon ginseng powder (obtainable at health food shops)
Juice the first 8 ingredients. Stir in ginseng powder and lemon juice to taste.

Vegetable Brain Booster

6 young carrots with their foliage, well-washed
1 head of broccoli, washed and cut up
1 or 2 young radishes with their tops, well-washed
Sprig of spring nettle, washed
1 gotu kola leaf, washed
1 tablespoon of alfalfa sprouts
A very small amount of the following herbs; basil, oregano, rosemary or their flowers

Juice of ½ a lemon
4 pumpkin seeds, liquidized in a blender with a small quantity of water and strained
Juice together the first 8 ingredients. Stir in the pumpkin seed liquid and lemon juice.

Medicine Juice

6 young carrots plus their foliage, well-washed
2 or 3 young leaves of cabbage, washed and cut up
1 or 2 stalks of young celery, well-washed
1 clove of garlic
1 sprig of thyme (small amount of flowers if available)
1 nasturtium flower or leaf
1 teaspoon cayenne pepper
Juice together all ingredients, and stir in the cayenne pepper.

Illnesses are often the result of an overly acidic internal system. Cabbage has soothing properties and is an alkaline vegetable, as is celery. These vegetables, combined with carrot, help to cleanse and remineralize the body.

Cayenne pepper is an effective internal cleanser. Too much can cause gastritis, so use it in moderation.

Longevity Juice

6 young carrots with their tops, well-washed
3 spinach leaves, well washed and cut up
4 young cabbage leaves, washed and cut up

1 small red pepper, washed with seeds removed and cut up
¼ inch ginger root, peeled and cut up
1 gotu kola leaf, washed
¼ inch piece of lavender, washed
½ sage leaf or 1 sage flower
Juice of ½ lemon
Juice together the dry ingredients and add lemon juice to taste.

Anti-Rheumatic Tonic

6 young carrots including their foliage, well-washed
5 or 6 leaves of young cabbage, washed and cut up
½ small red pepper (capsicum), washed, seeds removed and cut up
1 sprig spring nettle, washed
¼ inch piece of ginger, peeled and cut up
¼ inch piece of rosemary sprig or a few rosemary flowers
1 sprig oregano or marjoram
¼ inch sprig of lavender
½ teaspoon cinnamon powder (available at health food stores)
Juice of ½ a lemon
Juice together the first 8 ingredients and stir in the cinnamon and lemon juice to taste.

Blues Beater

6 young carrots with their tops, well-washed
2 beetroots with tops, washed and scrubbed
5 or 6 leaves of young cabbage leaves, washed and cut up
½ a small red pepper, washed, seeds removed and cut up
3 or 4 of the following flowers: geranium (of the Pelargonium species), basil, lemon balm, lavender, thyme and borage. If the flowers are unavailable, use a few leaves and stalks.
¼ inch piece of ginger, peeled and cut up
½ teaspoon cumin powder (available at health food stores)
Juice of ½ a lemon to taste
Juice together the first 6 ingredients. Stir in cumin powder and lemon juice to taste.

Spring Surprise

3 beetroots with their tops, washed and scrubbed
1 handful of broccoli florets
2 tomatoes, washed and cut up
1 small red pepper (capsicum), washed with seeds removed
1 clove of garlic, peeled
¼ inch piece of ginger, peeled and cut up
1 small bunch spring nettle, washed (wear gloves!)
1 or 2 dandelion leaves
½ teaspoon kelp

Juice of ½ a lemon

Juice the first 8 ingredients. Stir in the kelp and lemon juice to taste.

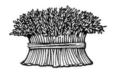

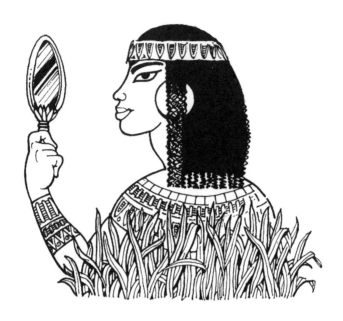

7

Green – Gold Beauty Saviours

Cosmetics made from plants, oils, mud, ochre and colored minerals are as old as recorded time. Knowledge of these natural hygienic substances still exists among primitive cultures such as the nomadic Fulani who are thought to be the original inhabitants of Africa. The Fulani are a branch of the Bororo who live south of the Sahara. These gentle and beautiful people continue to live their lives according to time-honoured traditions. Socially graceful, the art of natural body care and make-up is of extreme importance to them.

Our cosmetic and medical roots stem from Egypt, Mesopotamia, India and even China, via the ancient Greeks. Egyptian medical/cosmetic papyri include references to many familiar plant substances. These include: barks, leaves, flowers and fruits – carob, fig, cedar and watermelon to name but a few. Of the flowers, the lotus was reigning queen. To the ancients, the lotus symbolised the crown chakra. Lotus flower is currently being used in tinctures for the alignment of chakra energy. Tinctures of lotus flower should only ever be taken under medical supervision as large amounts can cause paralysis.

Among the cereal grasses, barley and wheat were also common medicinal and cosmetic aids.

Beauty and Balance.

Nature provides us with all we need to care for ourselves. The 'wild' is not chaotic and disordered. Our earth is a beautiful jewel. Mother Earth wishes to see us dance in her woods and glades and lead *balanced*, meaningful lives. Scientific and medical evidence supports the view that balance and moderation in eating, drinking, stress management, exercise and spiritual values are what is needed to keep us healthy.

Healthy blood with an ideal pH value of 7.35 – 7.45 suggests that at least 75% of the food we eat should be alkaline forming if we are to remain in proper balance (1). After absorption and assimilation, this food will leave an alkaline ash. Good alkalizing foods are sprouts such as alfalfa, clover, cabbage, mustard; most organically grown fruits and greens (preferably in their natural state); millet and almonds. Wheatgrass is one of the most dynamic alkalizers that we have available. The modern life that we experience does not always reflect a balance. Unbalanced eating/drinking, stress, lack of personal joy and spiritual/religious aspirations can wreak havoc on the body, mind and spirit.

Wheatgrass – A Beauty Aid

Derivatives of wheat are currently being used in many leading cosmetic houses because of their antioxidant and vitamin E properties. These and other properties in wheat, and especially in wheatgrass, are powerful allies in the fight against aging skin.

A superbly gentle skin cleanser, wheatgrass is also a wonderful toner. When applied regularly onto the skin it will eventually fade blemishes and sunspots. It stimulates the growth of healthy new skin and 'tightens' older skin. Quickly absorbed by the skin, it leaves it feeling silky smooth and gives it a golden glow.

As much as 60% or more of wheatgrass material may be absorbed by the skin. Fresh wheatgrass has a higher medicinal value than in the dried form because enzymes and other vital nutrients are still intact. It also contains carotene, which, according to Ann Wigmore in *The Wheatgrass Book*, is one of the substances that prevents oils from becoming free radicals while plants are alive. Scientific research shows that giving animals extra carotene from food sources or in foods, had a major protective effect against the formation of free radicals in the animals' tissues. Dried wheatgrass powder has a higher protein value than when it is fresh. Sunburnt or radiated skin benefits from the application of wheatgrass pulp; it is soothing and has excellent healing powers. Because of its stimulating qualities, wheatgrass may bring blood to the surface of the skin, so it is not advisable to use after surgery.

How to Use Wheatgrass Pulp

Juice wheatgrass in a wheatgrass juicer and use the pulp or resulting residue on the skin. If it appears too dry, mix a little of the extracted juice back into it.

An ordinary blender has certain advantages over a wheatgrass juicer in that raw honey, flowers, fresh herbs and purified water can be blended in at the same time. Drink the juice (according to your detoxifying capabilities) and use the pulp as a face and skin food. Take a small handful of pulp and dab onto the face and all over the body. Roll firmly over rough areas such as elbows and knees. Wheatgrass pulp also benefits the health of gums and teeth. Simply shape a small handful of wheatgrass pulp into a loaf-form and cover your top or lower teeth and gums with it. Leave in for 20 minutes or longer.

For additional nutrition and beauty benefits, use flowers and raw honey too!

Flower Power

The soul or 'eye' of the plant lies within its flower. From our fellowship with flowers comes respect and harmony. Only ever pick what is absolutely essential.

Flowers have a high vibrational power and energy, and respond immediately to the forces of nature. Dandelion flowers, for example, open for a few hours in the day when the sun is optimal for its well being. Flowers picked during this optimal time will give you the enhanced qualities of the plant. Most flowers being used for medicinal or cosmetic purposes are best picked at the hottest time of the day.

Potent Flower Beautifiers

Rosemary – has tonic and antiseptic properties. Good for removing freckles and wrinkles.

Yarrow – is cleansing, astringent and protective. Excellent treatment for slow-healing wounds. Use only for short periods of time as it may irritate the skin.

Nasturtium – has antiseptic and stimulating qualities. Beneficial acne treatment. Smoothes rough elbows and heels. Contains Vitamin E.

Peppermint and Catmint – Their cooling properties soothe inflamed skin. They also perk up tired-looking skin.

Basil – invigorates the skin and is used to stimulate slow-healing wounds. Keeps mosquitoes and other unfriendly creatures away!

Lavender – A gentle cleansing tonic, anti-inflam matory and a healer for delicate skin. Used in the perfume industry for its fresh scent.

Sage – is a potent astringent and antiseptic with anti-fungal properties. Has a delightful uplifting fragrance. Do not use before going to bed because of its stimulating effect.

Rose – The petals soothe inflamed skin and are antiseptic. A great beautifier.

Geranium (Pelargonium species) – They are very fragrant and soothe tight skin and emotions.

The Power of Honey

Honey is the end product of the bee's foray into the flower kingdom. Bees are drawn to airborne pollens, substances produced by the anthers of seed-bearing plants,

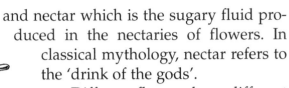

and nectar which is the sugary fluid produced in the nectaries of flowers. In classical mythology, nectar refers to the 'drink of the gods'.

Different flowers have different properties, and bees go in search of food that will give their honey qualities vital to the well-being of the hive. Antiseptics are found in rosemary, sage, thyme and lime flowers. Dandelion, which is one of their favorites, contains rubber (caoutchouc), pro-vitamin A, and vitamins B and C, a glycoside, sterols, and amino acids. Its flowers also contain carotenoids and triterpenes.

Besides its pollen, one of the important constituents of raw honey is propolis.

Doctors at the National Heart and Lung Institute in London have been investigating bee propolis for use in the fight against antibiotic-resistant hospital infections. "Bees create propolis by chewing the bark and buds of firs and poplars and mixing it with secretions from their glands to create a sticky substance. Scientists say it makes the hive more sterile than a modern hospital". (The Telegraph, London. Article written by Victoria Macdonald entitled, "Nun Zaps Alzheimer's with Bees' Own Muti.") Propolis has also been found to aid patients with certain degenerative brain disorders such as Alzheimer's and progressive dementia.

Raw honey has many advantages over heated honey insofar as the enzymes and other valuable properties are kept intact. Honey contains an active ingredient called tryptophane which increases seratonin levels in your brain. Seratonin, a 'feel good' hormone, has a restful effect on the body and will help you get a good nights sleep!

For Instant Glamor

Make a wheatgrass, flower and honey pack for face and body.

1 tray wheatgrass, cut off at roots and washed

3 cups purified or bottled spring water

1 tablespoon raw honey

Flowers in season, e.g. 6 rosemary, 1 yarrow (only in emergencies, and for short periods), 2 – 3 nasturtiums, 2 – 3 mints, 6 – 8 basil, 1 flowering head of lavender, 1 rose, a few flowers each of geranium and sage. Sage is toxic when used in large quantities over a long period of time.

In a blender, liquify all the above ingredients for 1 – 2 minutes – strain. Drink according to your detoxifying capabilities and use the pulp as an ideal skin food.

Break off a walnut sized piece of wheatgrass pulp and start off by dabbing this wad over the face, neck, chest, arms, hands, fingers, nails, etc. – all over the body. Pay attention to feet and toes.

The honey will make you feel sticky. Persevere for at least 20 minutes. Now use a good cold-pressed cleansing oil such as vitamin E (recipe for Wheatgrass oil later on in the chapter) or sesame oil and apply to the whole body. Find a warm, protected spot and allow the oil to soak in for a few minutes. Use an old towel and remove all excess wheatgrass, flower, honey and oil residue. A brisk action will stimulate the skin. This remedy will give you a quick lift as it:

* cleanses the skin by filtering out impurities
* improves the circulation
* 'flushes' the skin
* has toning properties and firms contours
* heals and rejuvenates
* gives the skin a golden glow with continued use

When you are using flowers as in body care and juices, be advised that you are opening new doors of understanding. Flower essences, even in the most minute quantities, are absorbed and can have definite effects on the emotional, mental and spiritual states, especially when they are used regularly. It may be helpful to start off by using one or two flowers and monitoring their effects before you move on.

Which Flowers to Start With?

One of the gentlest flowers to use in home treatment is *lavender*. Lavender benefits all skin types. It has antiseptic properties and has a soothing effect on the skin. A good treatment for acne and skin inflammations, it also encourages the development of new skin. A few drops of lavender aroma therapy oil may be used on burns for pain relief and healing. Lavender has a quietening effect on the emotions and helps to relieve panic and anxiety. Geranium (Pelargonium species) may irritate sensitive skin. To know how it will effect you, prepare a small amount. Liquify one geranium flower with a handful of wheatgrass (both gently washed) in ½ cup of purified water, strain, remove excess liquid, and place a very small amount of this pulp onto the gauze section of a sticking plaster. Apply to the inner arm (between elbow and wrist) and leave on for approximately 24 hours, by which time you will know how it will react on your body.

Geranium (Pelargonium species), can be used for dry or greasy skin conditions. It has a cleansing effect on greasy skin and is a good treatment for eczema as it helps to unblock pores. Geranium also combats inflammation and soothes the skin. Its astringent properties make it a beneficial treatment for a variety of illnesses including diarrhoea, PMS, fluid retention and circulatory problems. Geranium has an uplifting and balancing effect on the nerves and mind and provides a silky balm for enhanced sensuality.

Easy to make first-aid beauty products

Wheatgrass tincture

To preserve wheatgrass's vital properties you may want to make a tincture. Alcohol has the ability to draw out the active constituents from plant material, and tinctures last for a long time.

Wash 8 oz. fresh wheatgrass and gently dry between paper towels. Cut the wheatgrass using a plastic knife. Put into a glass vessel with 1 pint of brandy or vodka. Stop with a tightly fitting lid. Keep this mixture in a cool dry place and shake once or twice a day for about ten days. Pour through a double muslin and squeeze this pulp so that all the liquid comes through. Leave to stand for 12 hours and filter again; you can use a coffee filter. Store in a dark glass jar.

5 – 15 drops can be used in a glass of warm water (purified or spring water is best) for a revitalizing face and body wash. A few drops may be added, along with a handful of wheatgrass, into a facial steam-bath. Gargle using a few drops of tincture in ½ a glass of warm water.

Rub a few drops of tincture onto receding gums, as long as you are alcohol tolerant!

Wheatgrass Oil

Fill a clear glass bottle with clean, fresh wheatgrass (loosely packed) and cover with good quality cold-pressed wheat germ oil. Cover, and allow to stand on a warm window sill for two weeks. Shake gently every day. Strain through a muslin. For a stronger effect, you can repeat the process, using a new batch of fresh wheatgrass. Wheatgerm oil, enhanced in this way, has tremendous nurturing properties and has many uses, including remov-

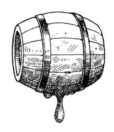

ing scars. It has a nutty fragrance, so you may want to mix it with a sweet-smelling oil.

Half the quantity of oil can be cold-pressed carrot oil. These oils can be obtained at health food stores. Make sure that they have not been extracted by means of solvents.

Wheatgrass vinegar

A ¾ bottle high-quality apple cider vinegar
A handful or more of fresh wheatgrass, washed and dried
Pour the vinegar into a pan and warm. It must not get too hot. Bruise the wheatgrass a little with a wooden spoon and place in the vinegar bottle. Pour the heated vinegar over and top with a cork. Stand on a warm window and

shake the bottle every day.

After two weeks strain and return the vinegar into its bottle. You may want to add some fresh (unbruised) wheatgrass and some flowers such as lavender.

When washing your hair use ½ cup of wheatgrass vinegar in your final hair rinse. It makes the hair shine.

Wheatgrass Hair Mousse

1 tray wheatgrass, cut at the roots and washed
For dark hair – 1 tablespoon rosemary flowers and 2 geranium flowers
For light hair – 1 tablespoon chamomile flowers and ½ a squeezed lemon
1 cup purified water
1 tablespoon cider vinegar or wheatgrass vinegar

Blend together all the ingredients in a blender for one or two minutes and strain through a coffee filter. Apply ¾ of this amount to dry hair and leave on, preferably under a shower cap for about half an hour. Wash the hair as usual, towel dry and apply the remainder of the mousse.

Wheatgrass Bath-Milk

Add 6 tablespoons of whole powdered milk with ¼ lb. dried wheatgrass and ¼ lb. dried lime blossoms or chamomile flowers. These flowers have a quietening effect on the nervous system. For a more stimulating action, orange or rosemary flowers can be used. Pour the dry ingredients into a plastic bag.

Add one or two tablespoons to the bath.

Wheatgrass Bath Salts

¼ lb. Epsom Salts
1 handful dried flowers
dried wheatgrass from 1 tray
glass container and stopper

To dry Flowers:

Fragrant flowers such as rose, lavender, sage, viola, jasmine or apricot blossoms can be easily dried. Pick blooming specimens in the morning sun.

Dry the flowers by spreading them on a newspaper or a large shallow basket and place this in a sheltered, sunny spot, preferably out of doors. Move the flowers gently every few hours. The drying process will cause most flowers to shrink in size. Repeat this process for a few days until the flowers are dry.

To make the bath salts, crush the dried flowers in-between newspaper with a rolling pin. Tear up the dried wheatgrass and mix everything together with the Epsom salts. Place in a pretty jar. To give the salts a stronger scent, add a few drops of your favorite aroma therapy oil.

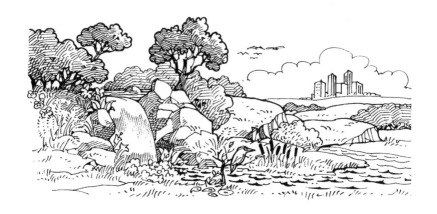

8

Back to Nature

Birds and bees beckon us to join them in their celebration of the earth. Sweet fragrances uplift the Spirit and take us back to ancient times when we lived in harmony with the forces around us. The Great Spirit continues to nurture us. Every day brings a new dawn with its promise for a better future.

Partaking of the new dawn in a spirit of gratitude will bring many blessings. Mother Earth, a patient teacher, guides us through many new doors of understanding as we allow her into our lives. Fields of grasses, flowers and herbs, grown in a spirit of ecology, will bring back the call of birds and other creatures of the 'wild' as well as nurturing our bodies, minds and spirits.

Above all, we must take care of each other.

Create your own Paradise

Paradise, a term of Persian origin, is traditionally considered to be a place which fulfils our aspirations for beauty in nature (1).

Wheat, which was first cultivated in ancient Mesopotamia, has great potential in such a Paradise. Wheatgrass, a 'super whole-food', not only benefits our bodies and minds, but also benefits our native soil in the form of wheatgrass waste such as the mat. The *wheatgrass-mat* is a valuable by-product of wheatgrass. This is the part which is not physically consumed i.e. when wheatgrass is cut off at the root, what is left behind is the mass of wheat roots which grow and entwine themselves in the bottom of the growing tray. These roots and the remaining soil have immense value for upgrading the soil, as mulching agents etc. This mat contains a wealth of vital nutrients. There are many uses for these mats in the garden. A healthy soil will produce abundant fruit and vegetables. Growing indigenous species of flora and fauna is always best!

The Wheatgrass-Mat and Soil Health

When young germinating wheatplants are grown in seedtrays, as seen in chapter 3, roots grow very rapidly in search of vital nutrients to build up a healthy wheatplant.

One can almost watch the roots in action. Place a 3 or

4 day tray of wheatgrass on top of a cut down wheatgrass mat (with its roots up). If only half the tray of wheatgrass is placed on the wheatgrass-mat, and the other half in ordinary soil, the roots exposed to the more nutritious wheatgrass-mat will show massive signs of growth, as much as four to six inches in a week.

When wheatgrass is cut down to the roots for use, for its juice or for the pulp, the mat with its developed root-system can be used to great effect for promoting the fertility of the soil in any part of the garden. To create a 'rejuvenating hot-bed' for some favorite plant specimens, dig out about 12 inches of soil within a diameter of about 24 inches. Place some cut-up sticks in your depression to encourage air circulation and place three of four mats roots up on top of the sticks. On top of this you could place a few oyster or egg shells. Layer with more wheatgrass mats and shells until you have a 'mound'. Water it when necessary. The mats will eventually dry out, but remain protective for a very long time. Every week or two add a few fresh wheatgrass-mats. If oyster shells are unavailable, mix one or two table-spoons of high quality kelp into a pint of water and add to your mound.

Super-soil

For the Earth to continue to nurture us and our children, there are many scientific ecological avenues available for re-building the soil. Here our greatest potential lies within our own gardens.

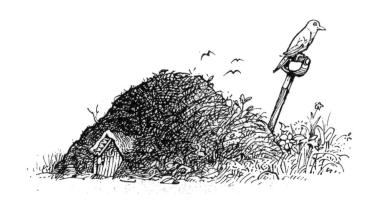

Its hearth and heart is the compost heap. This biological recycling centre is charred rich black in colour, moist and teeming with earthworms. It has the smell of a clean forest, warm and woody. Large and small birds will flock to it and scavenge upon it.

For those without a garden, re-cycling of soil can be done indoors, such as in a basement, by using a special composting bin.

Everyone can be involved in composting to some extent. Those who choose to participate will enhance their ecological consciousness and engender a healing energy. Wheatgrass can be intensively grown on a small-scale. So can many everyday plants, flowers and benefical weeds.

Harmonious living expert Bill Mollison has devised agricultural methods termed 'Permaculture'. Within this system one can grow trees, shrubs, vegetables, fungi, weeds and root systems on a sustainable, multi-crop basis.

To find out how to create a 'species-rich' garden, read *Introduction to Permaculture*, published by Tagari. Also included are, 'strategies for land access', 'business structures', and 'regional self-financing'.

Growing Herbs to Benefit the Earth and ourselves

As adjuncts to your wheatgrass therapy, the following herbs have great healing potential. They also benefit the soil by adding nutrients and helping the soil to 'breakdown'.

Yarrow

Yarrow, one of our foremost healing plants, was used by many ancient cultures for its magical powers. The sticks used in the I Ching were made from specially cultivated yarrow stems. The plant is named after the Greek hero Achilles, who treated his soldiers with the flower and leaf after the Trojan war.

Native to Europe and Asia, it grows throughout the world in hedgerows, fields and lanes. Soft, feathery leaves come off a stem which is generally straight, hard and strong. A profusion of white, pink or mauve flowers come out in spring and summer.

Yarrow is a 'sun-worshipper'. However, it will tolerate some light shade. This powerful herb will ensure the health of surrounding plants because of its strength and vitality. Its vivacity rubs off on surrounding plants to foster good health.

According to holistic practitioner and author, Susanne Fischer-Rizzi, *Complete Aromatherapy Book*, Sterling Publishing Co., Inc., 1990, yarrow has a balancing effect on the mind and spirit. It also supports intuitive energies and opens awareness to universal dynamism, so it benefits humans too!

Propagation and Harvesting

Buy a few rhizomes from your horticulturist. A rhizome is a thick horizontal underground stem. Its buds develop into new plants and can be divided. Water regularly, until the plant is well established. If planting by seed, germination takes between 10 – 14 days.

Yarrow makes a superb edging plant (it can grow to about 3 feet high). Leaves can be used all year while the flower has its strongest value at the end of summer. Leaves and flowers dry well.

Medicinal

* Antiseptic
* Anti-inflammatory
* Diuretic

* Beneficial for treating haemorrhoids
* Cleanses the blood and strengthens its flow – useful in the treatment of rheumatism and arthritis
* Yarrow has a calming effect on the system

In conjunction with lemon balm, yarrow is helpful in treating menopausal problems:

Add 1 or 2 sprigs of lemon balm to a quarter cup of yarrow; flowers and leaves. Pour 1 cup of boiling water over it and let it stand for a few minutes.

A powerful herb, yarrow may cause skin irritation when treated areas are exposed to the sun.

Comfrey

This 'miracle' herb is a 'hydroholic' that loves the sun and rich soil. It will thrive in a poorly drained area of the garden. Its 10 foot long taproots raise minerals from deep within the soil.

Comfrey is loved by farmers who plant it as a first crop in order to break-up difficult soil. When the plant has matured, it is cut back and returned to the earth in order to further improve it. Comfrey contains vitamins and minerals which include vitamins A, B and C. It also contains the minerals calcium, phosphorous and potassium. The high mineral content in the leaf has made it a popular animal feed.

Comfrey also contains allantoin, which encourages cell division and healing.

Propagation and Harvesting

Divide pieces of root and keep moist until well-established. Space them about 24 inches apart. Comfrey will grow to a height of 1 – 2 feet. You can pick fresh comfrey leaves anytime, except when it dies back in winter.

Medicinal

* Astringent
* Anti-inflammatory
* Comfrey contains emollient substances which soothe the skin and may help to heal scars

For sore joints, rough skin and sprains, pound a few clean leaves on a wooden chopping board until dark green in colour and gelatinous. Spread on a cotton gauze bandage and apply to the effected area. The comfrey hardens which may help to 'set' an injury such as a sprain. Re-apply daily for a few days.

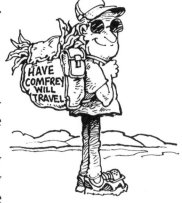

Cosmetic

Comfrey makes a good skin-softening agent. Leaves can be infused in the bath.

Use comfrey internally only when strictly necessary, as it may contain substances harmful to the liver.

It's usage can also encourage rapid cell division which can be detrimental if cancer is present.

Dandelion

Dandelion is often found growing in riverine areas. Its puffballs are known to children who make wishes by blowing them. In French, Dandelion means 'tooth of lion', a reference to its leaf which has sharp indentures. "The vitamin A content of dandelion exceeds all the store-bought greens by at least four times," says Victor Kulvinskas in *Survival into the 21st Century*.

Propagation and Harvesting

Dandelion is a perennial and will take root in many gardens. It likes nitrogen-rich soils. Roots, leaves and flowers have many medicinal uses and may be picked anytime anywhere.

Medicinal

Dandelion is used successfully in treating a range of illnesses, including: certain urinary infections, prostate problems and water retention. The leaves contain beneficial diuretic substances to help relieve sluggishness of the liver and cellulite accumulation. Dandelion also supplies the alkaline mineral potassium which can be lost to the system through increased urination.

Furthermore:

* It increases insulin secretion in the pancreas and is useful for the treatment of low blood sugar and diabetes.
* It cleanses the blood. Its tonic action increases the removal of toxic waste through the kidneys.
* Dandelion stimulates the release of bile which has a cleansing action on the liver and is a good remedy for sluggishness of the liver.
* Dandelion leaves may help to eliminate uric and other acids. It is useful in the treatment of rheumatism and arthritis.
* It enhances digestion and its root is mildly laxative.

The cultivation of herbs and plants is greatly improved with the use of high quality compost in conjunction with the previously mentioned wheatgrass mats. This combination, or even just using the healthy mats, is the stuff that the best 'mulching' materials are made from. Exploring and utilizing the secrets of soil dynamics is a science still to be developed. It seems certain though, that when properly used, the nutrients contained in the compost and the mats nourish the plants' root-systems. Water and nutrients are 'locked-in', a factor which encourages superior growth and vigor. The use of these mats as mulching materials have the added advantage of discouraging weed-growth!

The science of soil dynamics is an important building block in nurturing 'lack-lustre' soil back to its former, fertile glory. But this is only the first step. Re-engendering the nurturing aspects of Mother Earth must impact on all her people.

A harmonious and happy future for ourselves and our children would make the effort worthwhile.

Become a Visionary and Release the Artist in You!

A visionary, through insight or intuition, accesses images that are sometimes radical and nearly always idealistic. A visionary is akin to a diver who plunges into the ocean descending to the sea-bed in order to retrieve treasures. Caskets of gold and jewels found there are brought up to the light of day, examined, and offered up for the benefit of humanity.

The psyche lies within our deepest nature and relates directly to the forces of nature (2). Nature as perceived by a visionary may be a pulsation of lights, colours and shapes working together in harmony and with the source of all knowledge lying 'within'.

We all carry within us a psyche and possess its inherent wisdom. It dwells in eternity. Some people have the ability to 'dip' into this pure energy easily and effortlessly. Others find it more difficult. Meditation is a focusing on that conscious energy out of which the entire universe is manifest.

Visualization

Visualize an earth glowing with a coat of healthy, indigenous grasses, flowers and plants. Fruit-bearing trees and plants nurture its people. Like modern day temples, healing centers use scientifically substantiated therapies involving grasses such as Wheat and Barley and other 'live-foods'. They work harmoniously with traditional and modern medicines. These ideal healing centres, with their wide range of educational, scientific and medical resources, improve health and implement structures for rebuilding the Earth.

Visualization Juice

For a visualization boost, blend together blooms of the Clary Sage and other plants together with wheatgrass. This wheatgrass and floral bouquet will also promote creativity! See chapter 5 for the recipe.

A new millenium *dawns* – may the Blessings of the Great Spirit nurture and inspire us!

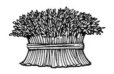

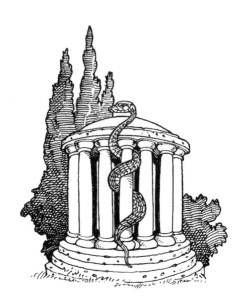

Addendum

Ancient Western Healing

The ancient Greeks, with their ordered minds and love of beauty and balance, made Health an institution. Under the guidelines of Hippocrates, health took on an important meaning. It involved the whole person, and sound mental, emotional and spiritual health were deemed as important as the health of the body.

Early seafaring ships of the Greeks traded with Egypt and brought back medicinal herbs and a wealth of knowledge. The Egyptians embalmed their dead and had an extensive knowledge of anatomy. They also had very developed ideas about the 'afterlife'. Egyptian heiroglyphic and symbolic writings were imitated by the 'pale skinned' people who inhabited Crete. Minoan Crete was the 'source and centre' of early Greek Culture. A clear sighted wisdom engendered by a thirst for truth was to propel Greece into the forefront of healing.

According to Greek mythology, Asclepios, the god of medicine and healing, originally came from Thessaly in Northern Greece. His father was the healing sun-god, Apollo, and his symbol was the snake. It was subsequently to become the emblem for healing.

One of his cults was in Epidaurus, an ancient state affiliated with Argos (ruler of the Peloponnesian states before Sparta). It was instituted at the end of the 6th century BC.

The Sanctuary of Asclepios was constructed on an even more ancient site, the Sanctuary of Apollo Maleatas. This site gives us a good indication of conditions within the Sanctuary, its ethics and methods of healing. Interspersed amongst the temples are baths, fountains, guest rooms, gymnasiums, a stadium and on the southern side, what is considered to be the most spectacular of all ancient theatres. The theatre, astonishingly simple and effectively designed, is a masterpiece of acoustics and was used to entertain guests with religious and moral plays.

Therapies used were water (considered to be very important), herbs and plants. Judging from surgical instruments which have been found, a sophisticated system of surgery developed in Epidaurus.

The most ancient temples of the sanctuary are orientated in an East-West direction. This suggests that the principles involved in worship are the same principles as in the worshipping practices of Egypt. (At Giza, the three pyramids are perfectly aligned in an East-West direction).

Was there a cross-over in religious-medical thought? Interestingly, during the Christian occupation under the Romans, many of the old structures were used, repaired and reconstructed. Important rituals were to remain. Baptism, which involved the immersion of the person in water, became an important step in the life of a Christian.

In Greek mythology, Demeter (Ceres), the grain goddess of the harvest, was believed to have been abundant to some, but not to others. In Greece's golden hey-day, however, a new humanity was forged. The disadvantaged (there was a huge population of slaves) found a new identity under Asclepios. Rich and poor alike often trudged for many miles over land and sea, to reach Asclepios' holy sanctuaries. When they were healed, they paid what they could. In the case of the poor, it was often just a rooster. The philosopher Socrates was put to death by being forced to drink hemlock in his prison cell – his last words were "Crito, I owe a cock to Asclepios, will you remember to pay the debt?"

Socrates, whom we know through Plato, (he never commited himself to writing) believed in the existence of an Absolute. "He held that Justice, for example, is not a matter of mere expediency, but as permanent and as invariable a reality as that two and two makes four. Such realities, or 'Ideas' as he called them, he regarded as the ultimate foundation of existence. They are fixed, eternal entities 'laid up', as he declared, 'in Heaven'; and it is only in so far as a particular act partakes in some degree of the 'Ideal' Justice, or as a particular object reflects the 'Ideal' Beauty, that either can be said to be beautiful and just. These 'Ideas', or realities, Plato would have us believe, are in a sense summed up in the uniting realities of Goodness, which is God – whether a personal God or a supreme creative force, he does not anywhere clearly define"(1).

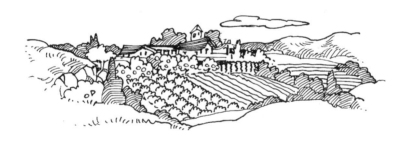

The Ideal Healing Center
Following the Ancient Tradition

Set in a scenic spot, preferably in the mountains and incorporating nature trails and scenic vistas, the ideal health centre is a restive and revitalizing haven. A serene atmosphere welcomes the visitor and provides the perfect holiday away from the modern world!

On arrival to the clinic complex, guests are medically assessed: blood pressure readings, blood tests and weight assessment. This information allows doctor and patient to devise a program to suit the individual. Included on the medical team may be naturopaths, accupuncturists, physiotherapists, iridologists, herbalists and other holistic practitioners.

Sophisticated facilities at the Healing Centre may include: hydro and oxygen therapies, gym and exercise equipment and recreational activities. Here, opportunities for the expression of the creative self includes painting and poetry, drama and music.

Workshops involving a holistic approach to living may include:

* Flower, grass and herb therapies
* Successful sprouting
* Wheatgrass growing
* Relaxation exercises
* Soil cultivation techniques

Healthy, organic soil ensures healthy crops. Ongoing, scientific testing of the soil is necessary, as is the testing of water.

In this environment, the advances of modern medicine work side-by-side with the gentle art of the cultivation of herbs, flowers and grasses.

The ideal Health Center has the potential to become

the Ideal Village. Resources in the form of medical health and education create opportunities to support the community. Here participation is central, such as: cultivation of food and medicine, manufacture of ceramics and basketware. Art in various forms, painting, music, dance and drama would benefit the community as a whole.

To Eradicate Poverty, Promote Education (for all) and Implement Health Care. Are These Goals Achievable?

A recent article, published in the Saturday Star, 3rd July, 1999 by Heidi Kingstone, entitled, "Short thrust to reach women in fighting poverty", explains current British policy on aid and development in third world countries.

The Rt. Hon. Clare Short MP, who heads the Department for International Developement, has a vision for a better world. Some of the Department's goals:

* To halve the proportion of people living in extreme poverty by the year 2015

* To target Primary Education for everyone

*To implement Basic Health Care

Short, in the article, says "The big new radical proposal is across-the-board development strategies for each country, using targets set by the local government. The UN has been part of the problem. You had an organisation to do health, to do children, to do family planning. All very worthy but if we're serious about this you can't have all

141

these organizations tripping over each other. They need to collaborate. Kofi Annan has really given the lead. He wants all the agencies to be housed together. We should have an agreed framework for how that country goes forward. Measurement is also important; we've got these targets, they're real. Let's measure year in year and see if we're making progress" (2).

A Proposal for Today

Ideally, science and technology should beneficially impact the lives of ordinary people, empowering them to live healthy, productive lives.

Some universities like MIT in Boston, MA are exploring a multi-fusion of knowledge that incorporates literature and art. Cross-linkages, which integrate important aspects of our lives, including our cultural heritage, can only be very enriching.

We may want to redefine other important issues and everyday realities which profoundly affect our lives;

* *Health*
* *Productivity*
* *Healing the land* (including the restoration of threatened species of animal life and plant forms)

By taking advantage of the latest in scientific research and integrating it with the ancient healing philosophy of Asclepios, we are in a position to target all three of the above directives.

In order to do so, an umbrella organization is needed to co-ordinate local bodies of health and environmentally conscious people to serve the needs of the individual and the community. This body would manage a broad spectrum of activities, including:

* *Funding.* A break down of costs is necessary. They would include running costs before profit, public relations, architect fees etc. Endorsed health products will help to attract sponsors from a large section of the business community, as will sponsorship of sporting events and gymnastics. Sponsors must know what they are getting in return.

Beleaguered countries should submit a proposal to the UN.

* *The management of medical staff.* Other staff would include gardeners and cooks versed in 'live food' therapy.

* *Cultivation of wheatgrass and holistic medicines*

* *Production of 'live' soil*

* *Beautification of the site*

* *Research, training and educational facilities*

* *Advertising and public relations*

Resources and Self-Funding

A handful of seeds can be a precious commodity. With care and knowledge, they can be transformed into healthy plants for food and medicine. When used resourcefully, these same plants have by-products which can be used to upgrade the condition of the soil. Wheatgrass mats, with their high enzyme, chlorophyll, mineral, vitamin and other nutrient content, greatly benefit soil-health. Great soil will grow healthy food and organic medicines!

The Production of 'Live Soil' is Profitable!

Live Soils, a report written by Eric S. Johnson, "The Benefits of Backyard Composting as a Waste Diversion Strategy in Boulder County" (July '96) says "On average, communities with backyard compost programs gain more than $3.50 in direct, quantifiable benefits for every dollar invested in the program."

Advantages of this system is that 'A-live' soils feed plants organically in a balanced way. Quality organic humus is always better and safer than chemical fertilizers and supports long-term soil fertility.

Healing the Land

In Africa, as elsewhere, much of the land has been scarred by erosion. It has been burnt, over-grazed and plundered of its trees and wildlife.

An important by-product of wheatgrass production is

the wheatgrass mat or 'green-manure'. It is valued for revitalizing 'dead' soil. It can be used on sites such as abandoned mines and areas of soil erosion. This material goes to work aerating the soil and introducing a friendly microbial population of earthworms. The soil becomes balanced, and it reflects a good acid-alkaline ratio, improving 'moist bulk density', and providing important nutrients like nitrogen, potassium, and phosphorous, in organic form.

In Africa, grasses, herbs and other healing plants are the 'stock in trade' of the Herbalist-Healer who may be termed a 'Sangoma' or 'Inyanga'. Plant collectors who supply traditional practitioners in Kwazulu-Natal sell approximately \$1 million worth of medicinal plants each year.

An article in the Star newspaper (SA), based on a study by specialists for the World Wide Fund for Nature (WWF) and the World Conservation Union, says that traditional medicine is a threat to many species of fauna and flora in eastern and southern Africa. The study found that traditional medicine is the most common form of healthcare in many African countries.

"Moreover, it is becoming increasingly important in countries such as Kenya and South Africa.

And in Lesotho, Namibia, Somalia, Sudan, Uganda, Zambia, and Zimbabwe, it is even an integral component of the state health system."

The sale of traditional medicines can help make this project self-fundable. Other opportunities for self-funding would be a modern clinic with trained and dedicated staff, gym facilities, spas and a food and health supply store. A well-run restaurant serving organic 'live' food in the form of green juices, sprout dishes, vegetable juices, seaweeds, etc. would also be potentially profitable.

The site, through proper ecological management, should be able to sustain indigenous flora, fauna and wildlife, thus attracting visitors, both local and foreign, to the Healing Center. The medical centre should be run entirely on scientifically proven techniques. In Africa, it should have links with organizations such as the Institute for Natural Resources in Kwazulu-Natal.

Eleusis – an Inspiration!

Eleusis, a little town near Athens, was the source of the 'Eleusian mysteries'. This is where Demeter, the Greek mythological goddess of grain, had her temple. Cicero, in about 100 BC, wrote "Nothing is higher than these mysteries. They have sweetened our characters and softened our customs, they have made us pass from a condition of savages to true humanity. They have not only shown us a way to live joyfully, but have taught us to die with better hope."

What these exact mysteries involved, we will probably never know. In ancient cultures such as Egyptian and Sumerian, cereal grains nourished not only the body, but the mind and spirit too!

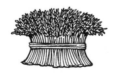

References

Introduction

1. *The Power of Plants,* by Brendan Lehane, McGraw-Hill Book Company, 1977.

1

1. *Lifearts,* by Evelyn de Smedt et al., St. Martin's Press, Inc., 1977.

2. *The Wheatgrass Book,* by Ann Wigmore.

3. *Survival into the 21st Century,* by Viktoras Kulvinskas.

4. *The Wheatgrass Book.*

5. *Survival into the 21st Century.*

6. *Survival into the 21st Century.*

7. *The Wheatgrass Book.*

8. *Oxygen and Ozone therapies* – www.oxytherapy.com

9. Dr Chris Barnard as quoted in an article entitled,"'Simple and effective', but not for Chris Barnard," in the Star Newspaper(SA).

10. *The Wheatgrass Book.*

11. *The Wheatgrass Book .*

12. Health Talk Magazine – an article written by Harry Rudolph and Prof. Willem Serfontein.

13. Health Talk Magazine, an article written by Harry Rudolph and Prof. Willem Serfontein.

2

1. *The Dawn of Man* by Steve Parker. Crescent Books, 1992.
2. *The Power of Plants* by Brendan Lehane.
3. *Africa Continent Revealed*, C. Struik (Pty) Ltd., 1980 by Rene Gordon.
4. *Egyptian Myths* by George Hart .
5. *ABC of Egyptian Hieroglyphs* by Jaromir Malek, "On the pyramidion of Teti, the god Osiris is called hnty imntyw (*khentey imenteyu), 'the first of the westerners' (imntyw is the plural form of the adjective imnty, *imentey, 'western' or 'the westerner', and the last sign is the triliteral tyw), referring to the role of the god as the ruler of the inhabitants of the west, i.e. the dead. The Egyptians located the realm of the dead in the west."
6. *Egyptian Mysteries* by Lucie Lamy.
7. *Egyptian Mysteries* by Lucie Lamy.
8. *Coptic Apochrypha* by E.A.Wallis Budge.
9. *Egyptian Religion* by E.A. Wallis Budge.
10. Good News Bible. Daniel 4.

3

1. *Aim* – Barleygreen and Herbal Fiberblend.

4

1. *Complete Aromatherapy Handbook* by Susanne Fischer-Rizzi, Sterling Publishtng Co., Inc. 1990.
2. *Survival into the 21st Centuary* by Victoras Kulvinskas, OMango D'Press, 1975.
3. *The Nature Doctor* by Dr. H.C.A.Vogel, Bookman Press, 1952.
4. *A-Z of Herbs* by Margaret Roberts, Southern Book Publishers (Pty) Ltd, 1993.
5. *Survival into the 21st Century.*
6. *Survival into the 21st Century.*

5

1. *Introduction to Permaculture* by Bill Mollison with Reny Mia Slay, Tagari Publication, 1991.
2. *The New Collins English Dictionary,*1982.
3. *Survival into the 21st Century* by Victor Kulvinskas.

6

1. *The Nature Doctor* by Dr. H. C. A. Vogel.
2. *The Nature Doctor.*
3. *The Tao of Health, Sex and Longevity* by Daniel Reid, Simon & Schuster Ltd, 1989.
4. URL/heinerman/organicbeetjuice.html.
5. *The Nature Doctor.*
6. Essential Magazine (SA).
7. Fairlady (SA), 4 August, 1999, an article written by Pam

Sherriffs.

7

1. *The Natural Way*, Recipe Book 2 by Mary-Ann Shearer, Ibis Books and Editoral Services, 1995

8

1. The New Collins Concise English Dictionary.
2. *Carl G. Jung in Man and his Symbols*, Aldus Books, 1964 - pg. 23, says, "our psyche is part of nature, and its enigma is limitless."

Addendum

1. *A History of Greece* by Cyril E. Robinson Methuen & Co. LTD. 1929.
2 Saturday Star, 3rd July, 1999.

Additional Reading

The Last Africans by Gert Chesi. C. Struik Publishers (Pty) Ltd, 1980.
A-Z of Herbs by Margaret Roberts, Southern Book Publishers, 1993.
The Illustrated Encyclopaedia of Herbs edited by Sarah Bunney, Chancellor Press.
Herbs and Aromatherapy by Joanna MetCalfe, Bloomsbury Books1992.

Complete Aromatherapy Handbook by Susanne Fischer-Rizzi, Sterling Publishing, 1990.

The Complete Floral Healer by Anne Mc Intyre, Gaia Books, 1996.

The Complete Book of Herbs by Lesley Bremness, published by Southern Book Publishers, 1988.

Larousse Encyclopedia of Prehistoric and Ancient Art. General Editor Renë Huyghe, published by Paul Hamlyn, 1962.

U.S. Wheatgrass Resources

Hippocrates Health Institute
General Info.: 1-561-471-8876 Reservations: 1-800-842-2125
www.hippocratesinst.com

Wheatgrass Juicers:

Sundance Industries/Wheateena
1-914-565-6065
www.noriv.com/sundance

Green Power International
1-888-254-7336
www.greenpower.com

Omega Products Inc.
1-800-633-3401
E-mail: omegaus@aol.com

Miracle Exclusives Inc.
1-800-645-6360
www.miracleexclusives.com

HealthWise
1-800-942-3262
www.hwhealth.com

Wheatgrass Growing Supplies:

Gourmet Greens
1-802-875-3820
www.gourmetgreens.com

Utah Wheatgrass
1-435-427-3245
www.utahwheatgrass.com

Fresh (Frozen) Wheatgrass Juice:

Hawkhaven Greenhouse Int'l
1-920-540-3536
www.hawkhaven.com

Evergreen Wheatgrass Juice
1-905-886-8090
www.evergreenjuices.com

Freeze-Dried Wheatgrass Juice:

Sweet Wheat Inc.
1-888-22-SWEET
www.sweetwheat.com

Other Wheatgrass Products:

Now Foods
1-800-999-8069
www.nowfoods.com

Pines International
1-800-697-4637
www.wheatgrass.com

Green Foods Corp.
1-800-777-4430
www.greenfoods

Green Kamut
1-800-452-5769
askgrassman@greenkamutcorp.com

Pure Planet
1-520-204-1806
www.pureplanet.com

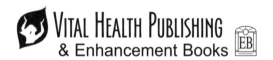

VITAL HEALTH PUBLISHING
& Enhancement Books

All Vital Health Publishing and Enhancement Book titles are available through your local bookseller or natural food store. If you cannot find a title, call 877-VIT-BOOKS or visit us online at www.vitalhealthbooks.com.

Distributed in the U.S. by Ingram, Baker & Taylor, New Leaf, Now Foods, Nutri-Books, Partner's West, Lotus Light and Quality Books. Int'l: AU: Gemcraft, NZ: Peaceful Living, SA: New Horizons, UK: Deep Books

34 Mill Plain Road, Danbury, CT 06811 (203)-794-1009

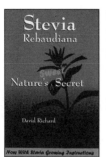

Stevia Rebaudiana
Natures Sweet Secret

David Richard

ISBN 1-890612-15-4 80 pp, $7.95

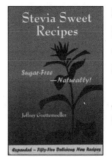

Stevia Sweet Recipes
Sugar Free Naturally

Jeffrey Goettemoeller

ISBN: 1-890612-13-8 196 pp, $13.95

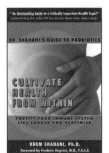

Cultivate Health From Within
Dr. Shahani's Guide to Probiotics

Khem Shahani, Ph.D.

ISBN 1-890612-42-1 164 pp $13.95

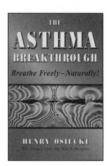

The Asthma Breakthrough
Breathe Free-- Naturally!

Henry Osieki

ISBN 1-890612-22-7 164 pp $13.95

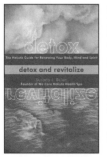

Detox and Revitalize
The Holistic Guide for Renewing Your Body, Mind and Spirit

Susana Belen

ISBN: 1-890612-46-4 120 pp $14.95

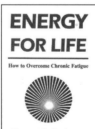

Energy For Life
How to Overcome Chronic Fatigue

George Redmon, N.D.

ISBN: 1-890612-14-6 248 pp $15.95